INPATIENT LABEL HERE

This journal was kept for:

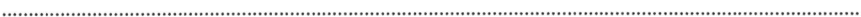

....

to document your ICU experience and to help
with your long-term recovery.

IF LOST, PLEASE RETURN TO:

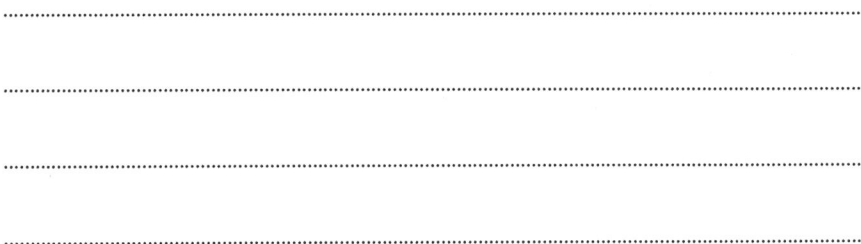

....

....

....

....

ÆMPOWER
PUBLICATIONS

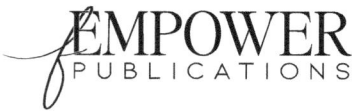

The Intensive Care Unit Journal

2025 fEMPOWER Press Trade Paperback Edition
Copyright © 2025 ACE PLANNING COMPANY INCORPORATED

Published in Canada, for Global Distribution by fEMPOWER Publications
www.fempower.pub | For more information email: media@fempower.pub

ISBN trade paperback: 978-1-998721-14-6

To order additional copies of this book: media@fempower.pub

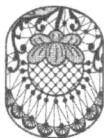

ADVANCE CARE &
EMERGENCY PLANNING COMPANY

PLAN FOR THE (UN)EXPECTED

THE
INTENSIVE CARE UNIT
JOURNAL

CREATED BY ICU PROFESSIONALS

Carly Hickey, R.N. & Michael Hickey, M.D.

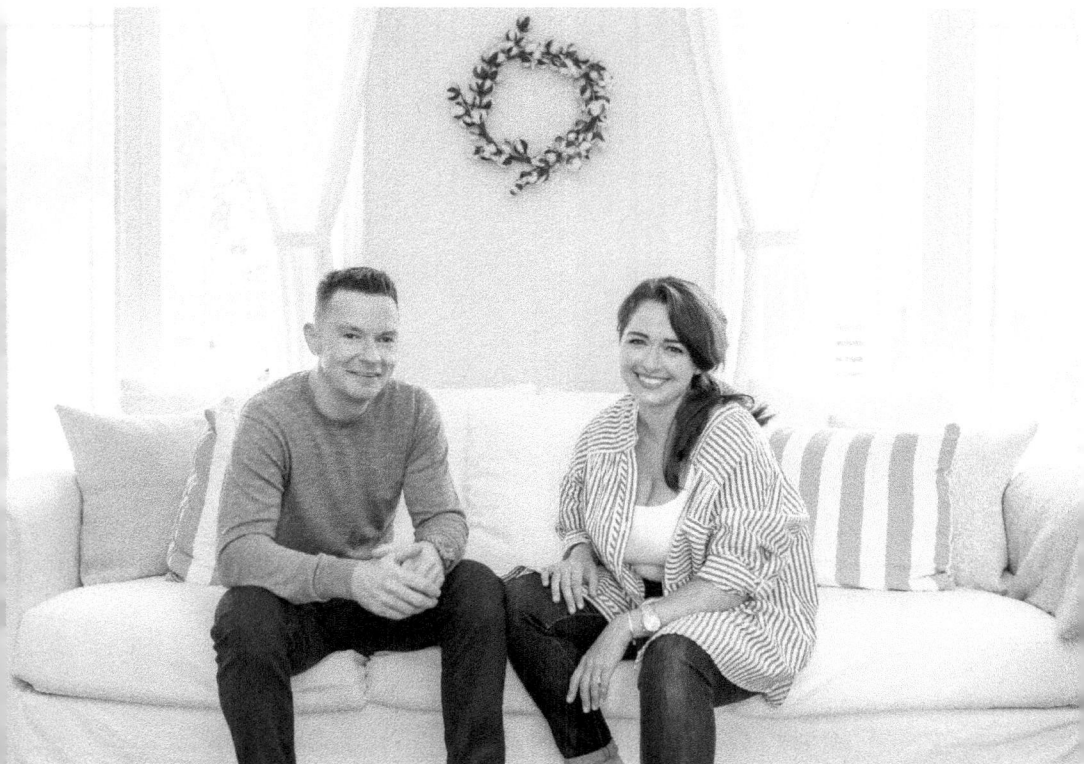

"The greater the love,
the greater the grief."

UNKNOWN

DEDICATION

This book is dedicated to two wonderful men who were taken too soon and two strong women who lovingly cherish their legacies.

Brenda & Bill Hickey (2015)

Tara Prendergast & Nick Polischuk (2016)

A MESSAGE **FROM THE AUTHORS**

If you have a copy of this journal, it likely means you or a loved one is receiving care in a hospital. This is a position no one ever expects to find themselves in and we truly hope for a positive outcome.

Over a decade of working in intensive care units (ICU) in Canada taught us one thing. Families cannot think clearly in crisis. This lesson was solidified when we experienced the ICU personally.

We set out to create this resource using both our professional expertise and personal experience as family when we lost two important family members in the Intensive Care Unit.

Following these experiences, our patient care was forever changed for the better.

- We listened better.
- We understood the intense grief of sudden loss.
- We understood what it was like to process information in crisis.
- We understood the importance of processing traumatizing events for grief healing.
- We realized we forgot details of our loved one's illness stories so many years later.

We took our professional and personal experiences and actioned them to create this resource for families.

This journal was created to:

- **Provide** clarity and comfort during a time of uncertainty and chaos
- **Empower** families with a role while their loved one is in ICU
- **Improve** the long-term grief recovery an ICU experience leaves on a family
- **Support** health care providers in providing an educational and efficiency tool to ease their growing patient care responsibilities
- **Document** a powerful story of strength, perseverance, courage and love into a legacy

Mike and Carly

H O W   T O   U S E   T H I S   J O U R N A L

This journal was created to help educate and support you—the family (or patient)—about what to expect during your ICU stay. There are two components to this journal.

P A R T   1 | T H E   H A N D B O O K

The Handbook was created to provide education to patients and families coming into the ICU so you feel more prepared and empowered during this vulnerable and chaotic time.

Many visitors and patients want to ask the ICU team questions but don't want to be a bother. This guide hopefully provides an educational starting point about the ICU environment, answering frequently asked questions and guiding decision-maker support.

P A R T   2 | T H E   J O U R N A L

The critical illness experience for patients and families makes it hard to remember details and the sequence of tests and events that occur. Many family members use phones or notebooks to take notes. A guided and structured specialized journal will optimize the note-taking process. The intention is for the family (or, if they are well enough, the patient) to maintain this journal to help the patient piece together memories of their critical care experience. This can help with critical illness survivor complications like post-traumatic stress injury and other psychological trauma.

This journal has been created by experienced ICU professionals who have thoughtfully incorporated answers to gaps in care expressed by families and patients. The goal is to hopefully bring clarity, efficiency and peace of mind to a highly chaotic and stressful time.

In the event the patient does pass away, the journal can serve as a tool to help remaining family process the sequence of events leading to the loss. Processing grief can take a long time for some families, and this resource can securely and respectfully chronicle that story.

HOW TO USE THIS JOURNAL

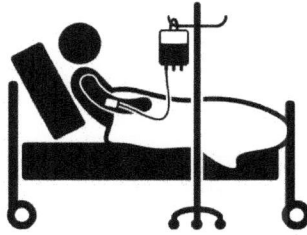

Your loved one gets admitted to ICU

↓

Have they started a journal?

YES ↓

NO ↓

Are they awake and alert?

How to get a journal

YES ↓

NO ↓

Patient can write in the journal themselves

Family member(s) keep the journal and update it regularly

Hospital gift shop
Ask the ICU Manager
Order online at aceplanningco.com
Use QR code
Amazon

WHEN THE PATIENT LEAVES THE ICU...

The family can give the journal to the patient when the time is right.

If the patient passes away, this journal can be used to process the experience while navigating grief support.

You can continue using the journal during the rest of the hospital stay.

→

ICU journals can be useful in post-ICU discharge follow-up clinics to support care and rehabilitation.

THE IMPORTANCE OF KEEPING

1   Research shows journaling can help patients and families **minimize the impact of post-traumatic stress injury** (PTSI) following critical illness recovery.

2   Journaling **helps families feel they have a role** in patient care during a time when specialty intensive care is provided by health care professionals.

3   A journal can help family members **keep track of details** during an emotional and chaotic time.

4   A journal can help **document the timeline** of the patient's journey and road to recovery.

5   A journal may be **used as a reference** for future illnesses and hospitalizations for recalling health events, medical details or identifying and connecting health care providers.

6   A journal can **serve as a keepsake** from a very difficult chapter in the patient's life to share with future generations.

AN ICU JOURNAL

7 Journaling can help families **feel more connected to the care team** by getting to know the name and roles of the patient's caregivers.

8 Journaling provides a **therapeutic outlet** for patients and their families during stressful times. It allows them to express their thoughts, fears and emotions.

9 Journals can be used as **a tool to improve communication** for large families where one representative can update everyone with accurate detail of notes taken in the journal.

10 Journals can **support note-taking**, improving recall of details and information.

11 Families will have a **record of care providers** to send gratitude or accolades to the clinical manager for care received.

12 Journaling may serve as a way to **organize thoughts and questions** for efficiency.

HOW TO USE THIS JOURNAL
DO LIST

✔ **Obtain consent from the patient** about their preferences for keeping a journal record of their illness.

If the patient is unable to communicate, ask the appointed substitute decision-maker for consent.

✔ **Let the care team know** you are keeping a journal for the benefit of the patient.

✔ **Find the organization's policies** regarding photo documentation of the patient's journey.

✔ **Securely store and protect this journal.** Though this is not a legal medical record, this journal contains sensitive and private health information. Don't leave it unattended.

✔ **Assign one family representative** to communicate between the ICU team and loved ones. Use this journal to organize your communications.

✔ **Place a patient label** in case this journal gets lost (if applicable).

✔ **Maintain hope** and remember that self-care is not selfish. Take care of yourself during this challenging time.

✔ **Let the patient decide when they are ready to review it.** You have put a lot of love and effort into keeping this journal for your loved one. Recovery can be a difficult process and time of grieving.

✔ It is helpful to **document procedures** that are common sources of hallucinations and nightmares that include: Tests (MRI / CT scans), restraints, urinary catheters, ventilator and suctioning.

✔ **Stay positive.** Include messages of caring, hope and resilience.

HOW TO USE THIS JOURNAL
DON'T LIST

✗ You may invite the health care team to write in the journal but remember that physicians and nurses have many responsibilities. **This is a family / caregiver led project.** This is a gentle reminder not to expect the health care staff to keep this journal updated.

✗ **Do not share this document electronically** due to the sensitive and private information it contains (e.g., via picture text or email).

✗ **Don't take pictures without** consent from the:

a) Patient

b) Power of Attorney for Personal Care

c) Immediate family members

d) Substitute decision-maker(s)

e) Organization and their policies

or if you feel this would go against the patient's wishes.

*Note: Organizational policies regarding inpatient photo documentation supersede recommendations within this journal.

✗ **Do not send picture texts** of entries from this document to large groups. Share information verbally whenever possible.

✗ **Limit access to this ICU journal** to the patient's closest family and friends.

✗ **Stop journaling if it becomes stressful.** It should be a helpful tool, not a burden.

✗ **Do not leave this journal** in a place where it can be lost. Ideally, bring this to and from the hospital with you to guard securely.

✗ **Avoid documenting only negative experiences.** Make sure to celebrate good days and progress.

TABLE OF CONTENTS

THE
HANDBOOK

PROFESSIONALS YOU'LL MEET IN THE ICU

INTERDISCIPLINARY TEAM

This term collectively describes all health care professionals within the the ICU care team. These professionals are described below.

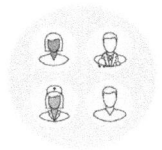

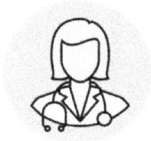

INTENSIVIST - PHYSICIAN

This term describes the Intensive Care Unit physician responsible for the care of the ICU patients. These physicians typically have specialty fellowship training in critical care medicine.

CRITICAL CARE NURSE

ICU registered nurses undergo thorough preparation before caring for critically ill patients. Though one nurse is assigned to the patient, you will often see many nurses working together to care for a sick patient.

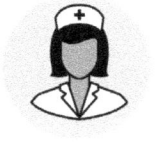

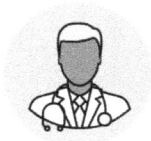

CONSULTING SPECIALIST - PHYSICIAN

The intensive care physician may need to call upon another physician with specialty expertise related to the patient's illness (e.g., Neurologist = Brain doctor or Cardiologist = Heart doctor). The intensivist may request a consultation from a specialist to help form a plan of care for the patient.

CONSULTING SPECIALIST - NURSING

While ICU nurses are highly trained in a range of specialty assessments and skills, sometimes, nurses may be consulted for a special procedure (e.g., PICC line insertion or Wound Care).

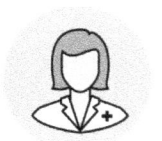

PROFESSIONALS YOU'LL MEET IN THE ICU

RESPIRATORY THERAPIST (RT)

The respiratory therapist works collaboratively with the team with specialized training in managing all aspects of the respiratory system. This person looks after the ventilator settings, getting patients extubated, vital in emergencies and all aspects of care.

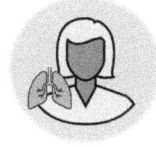

PHARMACIST

The role of the pharmacist is to recommend medications and drug doses, coordinate delivery or medication on schedule to the unit and screen for drug interactions. Ensuring we are prescribing antibiotics correctly is another mandate of their role (called antibiotic stewardship).

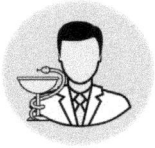

REGISTERED DIETITIAN (RD)

Critical illness is demanding on the body and nutrition is vital for recovery. The RD is a vital resource to ensure we are starting and stopping artificial feeding, as well as meeting caloric requirements for the patient. If the patient cannot be fed through a special tube in their nose or mouth, the RD may recommend nutrition through a vein called TPN.

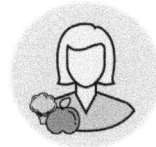

SOCIAL WORKER

Unexpected illness is very stressful for families and often reveals logistical issues that families need help sorting. The ICU social worker provides emotional support, helps families navigate medical decisions, coordinates care with the community, and connects patients with resources like counseling or financial assistance. They ensure patients and families have the support they need during difficult times in ICU.

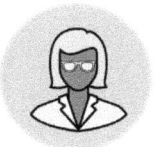

PHYSIOTHERAPIST

The physiotherapist helps patients in the ICU with physical rehabilitation, including exercises to improve mobility, breathing and overall function and strength. They also prevent complications like muscle weakness and assist with early mobilization to promote recovery.

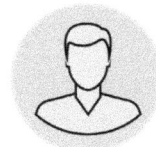

PROFESSIONALS YOU'LL
MEET IN THE ICU

SPIRITUAL CARE

Patients come from all walks of life and as such, religious and spiritual care is integral to caring for an individual holistically. ICUs have spiritual care leaders that can coordinate blessings, ceremonies and other observations relevant to top quality patient care.

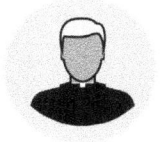

SUPPORT PERSONNEL (PCA / PSW)

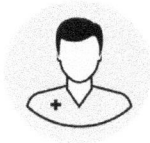

With a variety of titles in different hospitals, most ICUs employ a team of support personnel to assist the Registered Nurses in completing patient care tasks. For example, repositioning a patient often requires between 2-4 people, which is where support staff are extremely helpful.

WARD CLERK

The ward clerk team is the heart that keeps ICUs running smoothly. In charge of most administrative tasks, they are a knowledgeable and valuable resource for families to help navigate task-based needs.

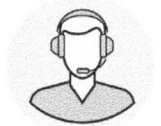

HOUSEKEEPING PERSONNEL

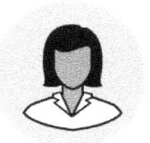

The housekeeping staff are responsible for maintaining cleanliness and sanitation in the ICU. They clean and disinfect patient rooms, equipment and common areas to prevent the spread of infections and ensure a safe environment for everyone.

PROFESSIONALS YOU'LL MEET IN THE ICU

CLINICAL MANAGER | ASSISTANT MANAGER

The clinical manager is the administrative leadership of the ICU. They have many responsibilities including staffing oversight, employee management and patient experience support, to name a few.

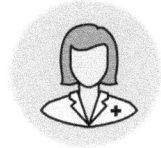

CLINICAL NURSE EDUCATOR

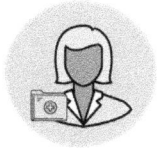

Most ICUs have educators who work alongside the clinical manager. They assist with onboarding staff and provide continuing education to maintain knowledge and skills for existing staff. Educators are also clinical resources to help nurses with patient care during their shift.

CHARGE NURSE

Most ICUs assign a leadership role to an experienced clinical nurse. Often referred to as a "charge nurse," they take on many responsibilities in supporting how an ICU is run. Listing only two of many examples, the charge nurse liaises with the management team for staffing needs and often coordinates patient transfers into and out of the ICU.

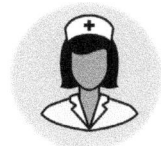

CHIEF INTENSIVIST

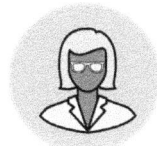

Every ICU has a group of intensive care physicians and the chief is the executive leadership of this group. They participate in patient care but also take on additional administrative tasks.

DIRECTOR, CRITICAL CARE

The clinical manager reports to the director of critical care. The director may also assign projects or tasks to the manager(s) that are in alignment with the hospital's strategic goals.

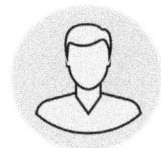

EQUIPMENT YOU MIGHT SEE IN THE ICU

CARDIAC MONITOR

A cardiac monitor is a medical device used to continuously track the heart's activity and vital signs. It displays the heart rate and rhythm, providing crucial information to health care providers about the heart's function. By monitoring the heart's electrical signals, it helps detect and manage conditions such as arrhythmias, heart attacks, and heart failure, enabling timely interventions to optimize cardiac function. ICU nurses receive specialty training in cardiac rhythm interpretation and are experts in this skill.

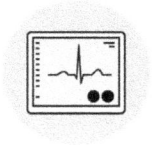

VENTILATOR

A mechanical ventilator is a life-saving medical device designed to help people breathe when they're unable to on their own. It works by delivering oxygen into the lungs and removing carbon dioxide, which is waste produced by the body. Ventilators are commonly used in ICUs for patients with respiratory failure due to conditions like pneumonia, asthma, or injuries to the chest or brain. It can also be used during procedures when the patient will get medication that might impact their breathing muscles temporarily. The ventilator supports the patient's breathing until their lungs can recover. Overall, it provides vital assistance to ensure that patients receive the oxygen they need to survive and heal.

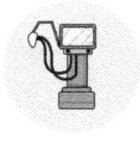

IV INFUSION PUMP

A patient in ICU will mostly likely need an intravenous (IV) infusion at some point. Controlled delivery of intravenous medications are provided through IV pumps. Most medications are prepared by the pharmacist or the ICU RN and administered according to the the Medication Administration Record (MAR). Medications are typically reviewed daily by the interdisciplinary team.

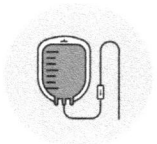

EQUIPMENT YOU MIGHT SEE IN THE ICU

HOSPITAL BED

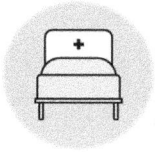

Patients will often complain about hospital beds being uncomfortable, but, ironically, it will likely be the most expensive bed they will every sleep in. Hospital beds have many functions and models are tailored to the patient (if applicable). For example, some have specialized mattresses that offset pressure sores; some can be positioned to help a patient walk upright out of the bed. Most have removable foot- and headboards.

EMERGENCY AIRWAY EQUIPMENT

As a basic safety measure, most ICUs require emergency airway equipment at the bedside, which you might find in the room.

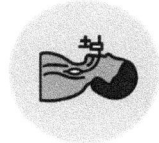

DIALYSIS MACHINE

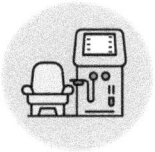

Kidney failure is unfortunately very common during critical illness. Patients may temporarily need support with kidney (renal) dialysis. Some ICUs have continuous dialysis (24h) and some have intermittent dialysis. You may see these machines being used for treatments on patients. Smaller ICUs or those located in rural areas may not have dialysis and the patient may need to be transferred.

ENTERAL FEEDING PUMP

When patients cannot eat food themselves, they may require nutrition through a tube in the nose, mouth or surgically created through the abdomen into the stomach. For any of these tubes, liquid nutrition is provided through an enteral feeding pump.

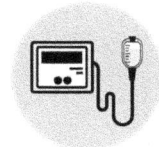

PATIENT LIFT

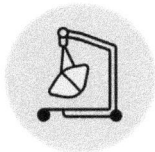

Patients who are sedated and unconscious require repositioning approximately every two hours (more or less) for mobility and to prevent skin breakdown. Patient lifts are required to minimize the physical demand on the health care team's bodies.

A GUIDE TO **TUBES AND WIRES**

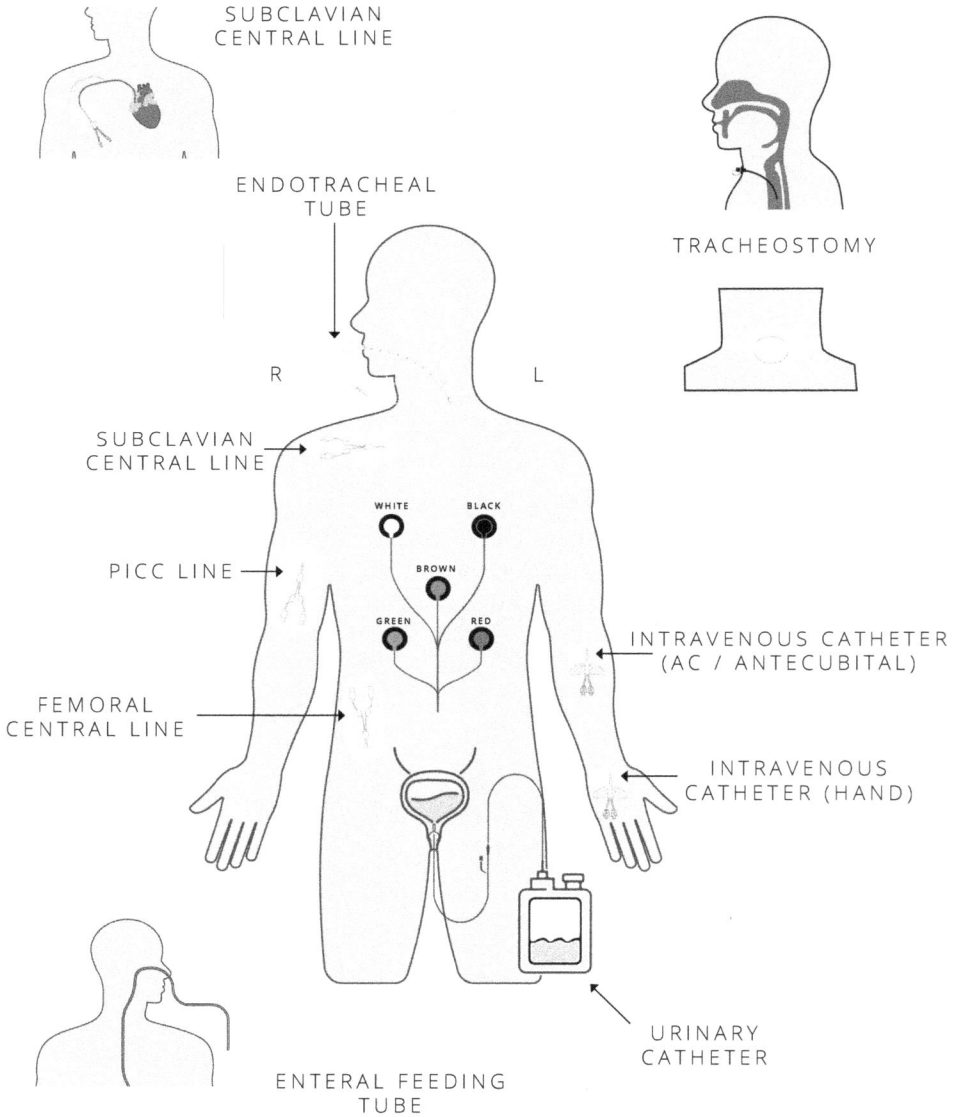

SUBCLAVIAN CENTRAL LINE

ENDOTRACHEAL TUBE

TRACHEOSTOMY

R   L

SUBCLAVIAN CENTRAL LINE

WHITE   BLACK
BROWN
GREEN   RED

PICC LINE

INTRAVENOUS CATHETER (AC / ANTECUBITAL)

FEMORAL CENTRAL LINE

INTRAVENOUS CATHETER (HAND)

URINARY CATHETER

ENTERAL FEEDING TUBE

NOTES

T H E   B A S I C S   O F
V I T A L   S I G N S

A NOTE ABOUT THE CARDIAC MONITOR

Bedside cardiac monitors are **a blessing** and a **curse**. It is a tool that provides the health care team essential real-time information about how the patient is doing. Nurses and doctors require hundreds of hours of specialty education and experience to master how to interpret and troubleshoot each and every vital sign presented on the screen. The curse is that they can really stress families out with the beeping and alarming or if numbers aren't quite right.

Each value also requires validation and assessment to ensure it is reading correctly before the team acts on it. Sometimes these monitors can produce false alarms. For safety reasons, the alarms must stay on (as the patient gets better or requires less monitoring, then the alarm settings can change and be turned off. There are organization specific policies so this may be different in your institution).

VITAL SIGNS

Vital signs tell us about how the patient is doing. When a patient is on a continuous cardiac monitor, the ICU team gets real-time feedback about what is happening in the body. The ICU doctor will often prescribe targeted ranges for vital signs to help guide recovery that is well thought out. Sometimes these ranges are different from what might be commonly seen on the internet. Medication is prescribed to achieve these targets and the ICU nurse will notify the doctor if interventions are needed.

Similarly, the high frequency of monitoring vital signs is often a frustration by patients and families and we understand where you are coming from. However, when a patient is really sick, it's important to monitor these vital signs regularly. As the patient gets better, the frequency of vital sign monitoring will decrease.

In addition to vital signs, we like to look what the patient visually looks like. We use both of these components to get a sense of how well or unwell a patient is. Some patients can have perfect vital signs but look very unwell. And some patients might have atypical vital signs but look good and report feeling well. Clinical assessment in addition to looking at the "numbers" (the vital signs and blood work) all come together when assessing the patient.

BLOOD PRESSURE

This is a measure of the pressure within the blood vessels that feed the body with blood. Blood pressure can be too low or too high, and either value if extreme can be life threatening. Blood pressure can be monitored with a blood pressure cuff, or continuously with a device placed in an artery. Nurses are trained to anticipate and act quickly to treat abnormal blood pressures to keep your loved one safe.

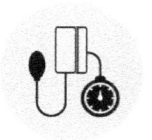

THE BASICS OF
VITAL SIGNS

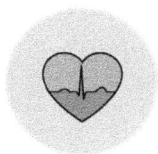

HEART RATE

This is a measure of how fast or slow the heart is beating.

RESPIRATORY RATE

This is a measure of how fast or slow the patient is breathing.

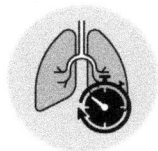

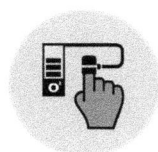

OXYGEN SATURATION

This is a measure of how much oxygen is bound to hemoglobin, a component in blood that delivers oxygen to the body. If the tissues of the body don't receive enough oxygen, the cells can die and this can be one cause of organ dysfunction or failure.

TEMPERATURE

This is a measure of the patient's body temperature. This can tell us if the patient might have a fever or cannot properly regulate their body temperature.

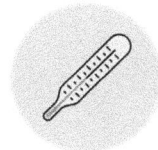

A NOTE ABOUT THE CARDIAC MONITOR

Having access to a pocket-sized search engine is a wonderful resource for looking up information quickly. It is common for families to get fixated on numbers and compare them to what they see on the cardiac monitor. Or they might feel a recommendation made online is what should be done for their loved one.

Rest assured, there are many reasons why a patient might have vital signs outside of the normal ranges posted on the internet. This is a gentle reminder that your clinical team have done tests and assessments on your loved one and gotten to know them better than the broad recommendations on the internet. The team also comes together to contribute their professional recommendations to create a cohesive care plan. Each specialist provides their own assessment or recommendation in an effort to move the patient closer to recovery without complications.

If something doesn't make sense, or you're worried something might be missed, ask for the team to explain their approach so that everyone is on the same page.

WHAT HAPPENS DURING AN
ICU ADMISSION?

DIAGNOSTIC
IMAGING

INSERTING
INTRAVENOUS
LINES OR
CENTRAL
LINES

BLOODWORK

ANY OTHER
PATIENT-
SPECIFIC CARE
NEEDS

MEDICAL
INTERVENTIONS
OR
PROCEDURES

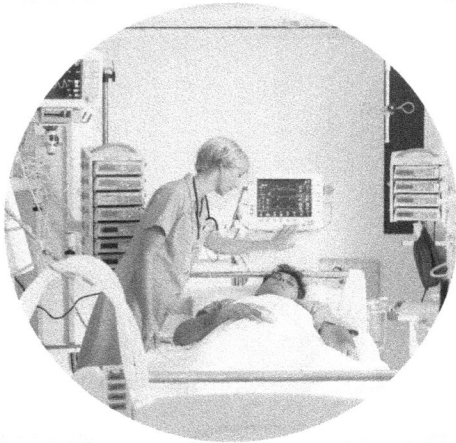

CARING FOR
PATIENT'S
PAIN, FEAR,
ANXIETY AND
EMOTIONS

UPDATING
FAMILIES

ORIENT FAMILY
TO ICU*

CONSULT
SPECIALISTS TO
ASSIST WITH
DIAGNOSIS AND
TREATMENT

COLLABORATIVE
INTERDISCIPLINARY
ASSESSMENT

* May not apply to every ICU: Depends on unit policies,
staffing availability and other emergencies in the ICU, etc.

ICU COMPREHENSIVE
ASSESSMENT

A severely ill patient in ICU will usually receive a comprehensive ("head-to-toe") assessment by an ICU nurse every shift. As the patient recovers, their care needs will change, requiring less intensive monitoring.

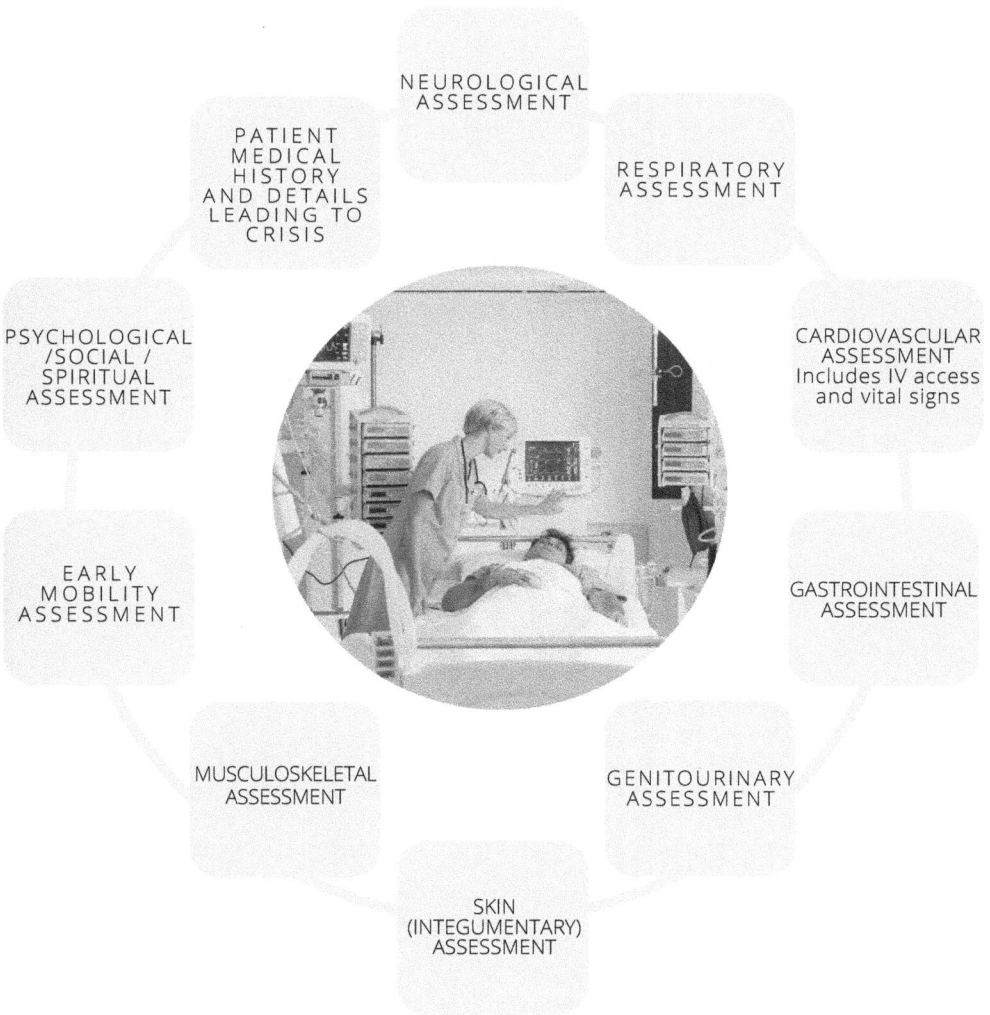

NEUROLOGICAL ASSESSMENT

PATIENT MEDICAL HISTORY AND DETAILS LEADING TO CRISIS

RESPIRATORY ASSESSMENT

PSYCHOLOGICAL /SOCIAL / SPIRITUAL ASSESSMENT

CARDIOVASCULAR ASSESSMENT Includes IV access and vital signs

EARLY MOBILITY ASSESSMENT

GASTROINTESTINAL ASSESSMENT

MUSCULOSKELETAL ASSESSMENT

GENITOURINARY ASSESSMENT

SKIN (INTEGUMENTARY) ASSESSMENT

CONTACT   DROPLET   AIRBORNE

ISOLATION PRECAUTIONS
IN THE ICU

START HERE

There may be a day you come to visit and the nurse tells you your loved one is under a new isolation precaution.

→

First...
Don't panic!

→

This is a very common procedure directed by the Infection Prevention and Control (IPAC) Team.

↓

A long time ago, hospitals were notorious for spreading germs due to the mobility of care providers and concentrated amounts of patients with illnesses within one building. Introduction of IPAC saved countless lives with excellent infection control protocols.

↓

Nurses are directed by IPAC to follow strict isolation guidelines if a patient presents with:
a cough
diarrhea
or other common symptom of a contagious illness

↓

Critical illness can cause many symptoms that initiate isolation requirements (liquid stools / diarrhea are the most common). Once testing comes back, isolation precautions can typically be removed.

L E A V I N G I C U

Leaving the ICU offers a unique experience for families and patients.

| HAPPY | UNSURE | UNCERTAIN |

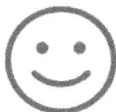

Sometimes families are happy their loved one is doing so well and are one step closer to coming home.

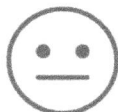

Sometimes families worry about not having around-the-clock care at all times.

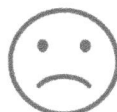

Sometimes a patient requires long-term end-of-life care best suited to the expertise of a palliative care floor or hospice.

The stress of a major illness is finally behind the patient and families can focus on recovery.

Families may have mixed feelings: Relieved their loved one is not suffering but sad they have died.

The thought of bringing a loved one home after a major illness is scary.

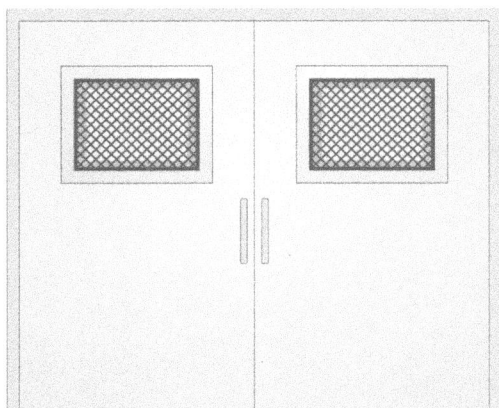

However you are feeling, **your feelings are valid**.

It is important to discuss these concerns with your care team to find solutions to help relieve anxious feelings. Some solutions may be available within the hospital or organization. And some options might be privately paid out-of-pocket expenses.

Peace of mind can be achieved through collaboration.

COMMON INTENSIVE CARE
PROBLEMS

Care in ICU is guided by strict adherence to the best-known practice recommendations for preventing complications and illness recovery. Despite best efforts, severe critical illness does come with unavoidable problems.

DELIRIUM

Delirium is an acute illness associated with low blood pressure, medication, altered blood work, breathing problems, infections, sleep deprivation and many other underlying causes of serious illness. Therefore, delirium is often seen in the ICU.

BRUISES

The lifeline of a critically ill patient is an intravenous line. Nurses continuously replace IVs if they expire or no longer are usable. Often times, bruising is noticed despite best efforts to minimize this outcome.

PRESSURE ULCERS / BEDSORES

When a patient lies in bed for several hours, the skin begins to break down compounded by poor circulation and malnutrition. Despite regular repositioning in many ICUs, bedsores remain a common consequence of serious illness.

SWELLING

Swelling is a common concern for loved ones as it is one of the most visual complications of serious illness. For more information on swelling, see the FAQ section.

INFECTIONS

Primary infections may lead to serious illnesses, while secondary infections can arise afterward. When the body weakens due to illness, vital organs failing, and the immune system weakening, it becomes susceptible to infection. Additionally, medical lines and tubes, though necessary for treatment, can also introduce infection risks.

PNEUMONIA

Pneumonia is often caused by an infection from viruses or bacteria that overwhelms the body. Various forms of respiratory support are used to treat the patient. Pneumonia may also be a complication from prolonged mechanical ventilation (e.g., endotracheal tube or tracheostomy tube).

ADDRESSING **CONCERNS** ABOUT CARE

The root cause of most issues that arise between patients, families and ICU care teams is unclear communication. If there is something you are concerned about, please address it early.

Spiritual care workers and social workers have a unique set of skills in communication and emotional intelligence to help support and navigate emotional difficulties that might arise.

Everyone is here for one reason: the care and support of the patient and their family.

REFLECT

Have you ever heard the saying:
"Don't make a permanent decision based on a temporary emotion."

Give yourself some cool-down time to think about how you are feeling. Critical care units see complaints and frustrations from family universally, and it does not always mean this is from poor care. It often is multi-factorial, with a large part being the weight of emotional grief and stress. Document your concerns in this journal. Talk about concerns with the care team.

If you decide there is an issue you would like to address, then decide who you need to talk to. Here is some advice:

If your concern is with a staff member, begin with addressing concerns with the person directly.

ADDRESS

You may also speak to the assigned nurse for the shift, the charge nurse and then the clinical manager.

Most organizations also have a department devoted to patient satisfaction to offer additional support.

FREQUENTLY ASKED QUESTIONS

F A Q s

WHAT IS AN INTENSIVE CARE UNIT AND WHY IS A PATIENT ADMITTED THERE?

An ICU is a specialty care area where severely ill patients, or patients requiring close monitoring, are admitted for care. Patients are admitted to this area for different reasons:

1. They are too sick for the inpatient unit(s).
2. They may require specialized monitoring that can only be done in the ICU.
3. They may require special medication or a special procedure that can only be done in the ICU setting.
4. They may come to ICU for monitoring after a procedure before going to the inpatient unit.

WHAT TYPES OF HEALTH CONDITIONS ARE TREATED IN THE ICU?

While the majority of intensive care units care for a wide range of patients, some large hospitals have specialty ICUs for specific conditions or organ systems. The most common example is the cardiovascular surgery ICU (e.g., CSICU / CVICU)

- Brain emergencies (e.g., stroke, seizure)
- Burns
- Chronic illness complications
- Head injuries
- Heart conditions
- Post-procedure monitoring
- Post-surgical monitoring
- Organ failure
- Overdose
- Respiratory (lung) conditions
- Sepsis
- Spinal cord injuries
- Stroke
- Surgical complications
- Trauma

F A Q s

While the majority of intensive care units can care for a wide range of patients, some large hospitals have specialty ICUs for a specific condition. The most common example is the cardiovascular surgery ICU (e.g., CSICU / CVICU).

Here is a list of some treatments:

- Antibiotics
- Antipsychotic
- Blood transfusions
- Cardiac monitoring
- Cardiopulmonary Resuscitation (CPR)
- Chest tube insertion
- Dialysis
- Early mobilization
- Extra Corporeal Membrane Oxygenation (ECMO)
- Intracranial (brain) monitoring and pressure
- Intravenous medication
- Intubation
- Mechanical ventilation
- Neuromuscular blockade
- Nutritional support
- Physiotherapy
- Palliative / Comfort Care
- Resuscitation
- Sedation and analgesia
- Temperature control
- Vasoactive medications to support blood pressure
- Wound care
- And many more

F A Q s

WHAT ARE ICU MEDICAL ROUNDS?

Every day shift, the interdisciplinary team gathers to review the progress of every patient and assign goals for the next 24-72 hours. The nurse will provide their morning comprehensive assessment (refer to the ICU Comprehensive Assessment outline) to the team, as well as report any events or blood work results completed since the last ICU round. A list of issues or concerns will be discussed with the goal of creating a plan to move recovery forward.

Typically the newly admitted patients, most sick or highest priority patients are assessed first, then patients awaiting discharge or transfer to the floor, and lastly, long-term stable ICU patients.

WHY HAS THE TEAM ASKED ABOUT INVOLVED FAMILY MEMBERS OR HEALTH DECISION-MAKERS?

When a patient comes to ICU, there is a high likelihood they may be in a critical state that prevents them from having the cognitive capacity or awareness to direct their own medical care. They may also have a breathing tube in place requiring sedating medication to keep the patient comfortable. A substitute decision-maker will be located by the ICU team to determine who will make health care decisions for this patient for the period they are incapable. This person may be legally appointed, and this title is dependent on the province, territory, state or country they are in. In Ontario, this would be the Power of Attorney for Personal Care.

Family members are called in to help provide a medical history, report of the events leading to the illness or injury, and any other relevant information that helps inform a plan of care for the patient. Estate and advance directive documents may be needed if they were completed. A final will is only needed after the patient has died.

F A Q s

The road to recovery in an ICU is paved with good days and bad days. It is important to celebrate the small wins and document the days of progress after the scary days. Families are understandably very upset when a patient has been doing well and has a setback. The road to recovery is a difficult uphill marathon, not a sprint.

WHY DOES MY LOVED ONE HAVE BRUISES AFTER IVS?

Emergency department nurses and intensive care nurses have a lot of practice starting IVs and are considered experts in this skill. Establishing intravenous access is a medical necessity to provide lifesaving medication to a patient and is important for emergency preparedness if suddenly the patient deteriorated. Some patients, particularly those who are elderly, frail and dehydrated, may have veins that are more challenging to place an IV in, resulting in additional attempts and bruising. Bruising may also be more likely if the patient has received a blood thinner. Causing the bruising is as hard emotionally on the nurses as it is for you, the family, to see it. Nurses never want to cause harm or pain. Please discuss any concerns with your care team.

WHY CAN'T I STAY DURING A STERILE PROCEDURE?

While this policy is organization specific and may not apply to all hospitals, the goal during a sterile procedure is to reduce any potential risk of microbial contamination whenever possible. The more people in a room during a sterile procedure increases the presence of microbes, as well as risk for contaminating the sterile field. Navigating a room with a sterile field takes experience and skill (ask any nursing student or medical student who has learned the hard way). Also, a sterile field typically means an invasive procedure is occurring where the provider needs the utmost concentration. Additional people in the room may cause distraction (e.g., family members fainting).

F A Q s

CAN FAMILY MEMBERS STAY WITH THE PATIENT IN ICU?

While this policy is organization specific, many hospitals acknowledge the value in the patient having an essential care partner. This is usually a family member who works with the care team to collaboratively provide care. Visiting policies are organization specific so check with your ICU to learn their policies.

It is very understandable why family members wish to stay at their loved one's bedside for extended periods of time. Loved ones don't want to leave the patient in case anything happens. Health care providers observe the burnout and exhaustion these long visits cause. Once the patient appears stable, we often encourage families to take self-care breaks. This might include taking a short break from the stress and noise of a hospital environment: going home to shower, change clothes, sleep in their own bed, and visit with their children or pets. They then come back feeling rested. Rest and self-care can significantly help with coping through stressful times. If you do not want to leave your family alone, you can switch out with other family members.

As well, the physical space in an ICU inpatient room is often very small to begin with. This space is further reduced with pumps and large equipment providing life support to the patient. Nurses are often providing care throughout the shift that may disrupt the family member's rest. As well, if the patient suddenly becomes critical, having space for many staff to easily move in the room is a significant safety priority.

As the patient begins to recover, many health care teams will advocate for protecting the patient's sleep hygiene by encouraging visitors during the day and preparing for sleep at night.

In most organizations, if a patient is progressing to end-of-life or palliative care, often the visiting policies are lifted to allow for family members to spend their last moments with their loved one.

F A Q s

Visitors never want to show up empty-handed. While cut flowers are always a kind gesture and help lift the mood in the ICU, it is generally recommended not to bring in flowers for different reasons. This policy is institutionally specific so check with your specific ICU to determine their policies. Other suggested gifts can be:

- Hand-drawn pictures from children
- Notes of hope and support
- Important (un)framed photos (photocopies)
- Spiritual or religious items (non-valuable: e.g., rosary, prayer books)
- Toiletries (per organizational policies—ask the care team what is allowed)
- Your quality time—spending time with the patient is a beautiful gift
- Meals for the patient's family
- Gift cards for the family for restaurants or coffee shops
- Group funding for hospital and illness-related costs

* Remember, items brought into a hospital have a high likelihood of getting misplaced so refrain from bringing in items with significant value or worth or original photos.

F A Q s

Swelling in the ICU is a very common concern for families visiting their loved ones. It can appear uncomfortable to the patient but most of the time does not cause additional pain (excluding severe and / or localized cases).

REASON 1 | FLUID RESUSCITATION AND RETENTION

When someone drops their blood pressure and / or has a high heart rate, we often have to fill their heart, veins and arteries (the circulatory system) with hydration (like blood products or IV solution) to help the heart work. Think of fluid in the body like gasoline in the tank of a car: your car cannot run on empty. Hydration is provided under close monitoring and supervision of physicians and nurses.

After a day or two, the fluid moves from the circulatory system and starts showing up in the limbs and body, specifically the hands, arms, feet, legs, torso and face in mainly dependent areas where gravity takes the extra fluid. Think of being on a long plane ride and how swollen your feet feel or seeing the line your socks make on your legs. Because the patient has been bedridden for many days, the fluid accumulates more and more. Full recovery depends on many factors, but swelling in many patients resolves as mobilization and recovery begin.

REASON 2 | INFLAMMATORY RESPONSE TO CRITICAL ILLNESS

Without getting too complicated (because doctors and nurses spend years learning about the complicated inflammatory process of critical illness), let's use a simple example of when you burn your finger.

When tissue is damaged, a signal is sent to the body saying it needs help to repair. The body's complex proteins and other chemicals rush to the area, causing redness, heat and swelling. This is an acute (short-term) inflammatory response.

This example is limited to a small burn to a single finger. Consider the inflammatory response the entire body undergoes during a serious illness or injury. This massive process releases biological components that contribute to fluid retention and swelling.

FAQs

REASON 3 | ORGAN DYSFUNCTION OR FAILURE

The heart, kidneys and liver all play a vital role in fluid excretion. When any of these organs are not working properly, fluid becomes retained. These organs are also highly vulnerable to injury and dysfunction from the inflammatory process that occurs during critical illness.

REASON 4 | MEDICATION

Certain medications used in the ICU can cause fluid retention and swelling as a known side effect.

REASON 5 | IMMOBILITY

Early mobilization is an emerging standard of care in many ICUs. However, some severely ill patients must stay in bed during the critical phase of their illness. For some, this can be days to weeks.

Fluid follows gravity and will settle in dependant areas, which is common for patients when they are in bed for a prolonged period of time.

REASON 6 | MALNUTRITION

Patients who have poor nutrition (e.g., seniors with little or no appetite), or have inadequate nutrition during hospitalization (e.g., patients who cannot eat due to needing breathing support or going for surgery) are at higher risk for swelling.

F A Q s

HOW IS PAIN MANAGED IN THE ICU?

Pain management is an extremely important aspect of care in the intensive care unit. Nurses and physicians are extremely experienced in pain assessment including verbal and nonverbal behaviors. Nonverbal behaviors may include:

- Facial expressions
- Grimacing
- Appearing restless or agitated
- Tension in the body (e.g., arms and legs)
- Sounds or noises (e.g., groaning)

Pain medication (also known as analgesia) is provided as a first line therapy to ensure patients are comfortable during and for the duration of intubation. These medications often treat pain and may have some sedating effects, which is why they are preferred over sedation-only medication.

Nurses often anticipate the need for pre-medication for painful procedures (e.g., like turning and repositioning or dressing changes) and have medication with a physician's order ready prior to these interventions. Some pain medications take effect quickly and wear off quickly, so multiple doses (according to the physician's order) may be provided.

A patient's pain assessment is typically assessed at the beginning of every shift and regularly throughout the shift (for post-operative patients, this might be every 15 minutes to every hour).

WHAT IS A "SEDATION VACATION"?

As patients gets ready to have their breathing tube (endotracheal tube) removed, and to provide the lowest amount of necessary sedating medications, the nurse will lighten the short-acting sedation medication every shift (or based on the physician's orders depending on patient acuity). Here, they reorient the patient and ask them a few questions to determine level of awareness and whether they are able to follow questions.

Not all patients receive sedation vacations due to severity of illness or risk of removing their breathing tube prematurely. Patients with brain injuries often require deeper sedation to rest and heal the brain. If you're unsure, speak with your team for clarification.

F A Q s

CAN MY LOVED ONE HEAR ME IF THEY ARE SEDATED?

We are never truly certain about what a patient can or cannot hear. Care is provided in a manner where the health care team always assumes the patient has awareness. The only exception to this is with confirmed neurological brain death where there is certainty of no awareness. Still, care for these patients is provided in a respectful, dignified, person-centered and life-honoring way.

As well, many ICUs follow recommendations of early mobilization and light sedation, further supporting the assumption patients have awareness while sedated.

HOW DO DOCTORS DECIDE WHEN A PATIENT IS READY TO LEAVE THE ICU?

The decision to discharge a patient from the ICU is a conversation informed by multiple members of the interdisciplinary team. Discharge parameters vary between hospitals so it is best to follow your organization's guidelines.

Commonly, the patient must:
1. Be weaned from all specialty intensive care medications
2. Must not require intensive monitoring
3. Have stable vital signs
4. Must be able to breathe on their own without the assistance of machines (some exceptions might apply like CPAP at night)
5. Must not require intensive 1:1 nursing care

F A Q s

WHY CAN'T MY LOVED ONE DRINK WATER OR EAT?

REASON 1 | HIGH RISK OF CHOKING (ASPIRATION)

There are many reasons why someone's swallowing may be impaired that may lead to choking. Consequences of aspirating stomach contents into the lungs can be catastrophic and potentially fatal. For this reason, the ICU team will take precautions to minimize the risk of aspiration.

REASON 2 | WEAKENED MUSCLES OF THE THROAT

Having a breathing tube in the throat can cause the muscles of the throat to weaken. This may make swallowing food and fluids more challenging, or potentially end up in the lungs (aspiration). With time, these muscles may regain their strength.

REASON 3 | FASTING

Many procedures require the patient not to eat or drink before a blood test, procedure, surgery or other intervention.

REASON 4 | POSSIBILITY OF PUTTING A BREATHING TUBE IN

If there is any suspicion the patient may need to be intubated (have a breathing tube inserted), the team will ask the nurses not to provide water or food. The reason for this is the risk of aspiration. While the breathing tube is inserted, the gag reflex may be stimulated, which could bring up acidic stomach contents that will damage the lungs.

F A Q s

WHY CAN'T MEDICAL DETAILS BE GIVEN OVER THE PHONE?

Canadian privacy laws are strict in the interest of protecting the patient. As such, health care providers must be particularly cautious in delivering sensitive information over an unsecured method like a telephone. It is very difficult to confirm the identify of the person on the other end of the telephone line. This is a result of learned experiences from ways in which confidentiality has been breached. Some examples include:

- Estranged family members disguising their identity to obtain information about their loved one when they should not have it.
- Media personnel disguising themselves as family to obtain an update on the patient's condition on a high profile media story.
- Patients not wanting their family to know about their health history.

For this reason, an excess of caution is exercised, with health information provided in person whenever possible.

WHY ARE THE NURSES AND DOCTORS FORCING MY LOVED ONE OUT OF BED?

Can you recall a time when you were really sick and you stayed in bed for a few days? Do you remember how weak you felt when you finally got out of bed?

This weakness can be far worse during a serious illness. Patients lose a lot of their muscle while lying in bed. When it comes time to go home, they are profoundly deconditioned and frail, which may result in other problems.

Helping get patients out of bed helps with cognitive stimulation, lowering levels of sedation, helping their lungs function in an upright position (as we are used to as bipedal humans), recruiting abdominal muscles, as well as so many other benefits. Tolerance for activity is carefully evaluated by the ICU team to ensure the patient can handle the demand and it will not worsen their condition.

To learn more about this, you can read about "early mobility in ICU."

IMPORTANT DATES

JAN	Mental Health Awareness Month		MAR	Pharmacy Appreciation Month
JAN	Alzheimer's Awareness Month		MAR 1st WED	**International Board Certified** Lactation Consultant Day
JAN	**Firefighter Cancer** Awareness Month		MAR 3rd WED	Dietitian's Day (Canada)
FEB	Preventative Health Awareness Month		MAR 8	International Women's Day
FEB	Psychology Month		APR	National Dental Hygienists Week
FEB 4	World Cancer Day		APR 1st TUE	National Caregiver Day
FEB 21	Mental Health Nurse's Day		APR 16	Advance Care Planning Day
FEB 28	Pink Shirt Day		MAY 1	National Physician's Day
MAR	National Social Work Month		MAY	Melanoma and Skin Cancer Awareness Month
MAR	Dental Assistants Recognition Week		MAY	Nurse's Week

IMPORTANT DATES

MAY	Paramedic Services Week		**SEP**	Pharmacist Month
MAY	Naturopathic Medicine Week		**SEP** 8	World Physiotherapy Day
MAY 5	International Day of the Midwife		**SEP** 13	World Sepsis Day
MAY	National Physiotherapy Month		**SEP** 15	Terry Fox Run
MAY 12	International Nurse's Day		**SEP** 25	World Pharmacists Day
MAY 19	World Family Doctor Day		**OCT** 15	National Pharmacy Technicians Day
JUNE	Brain Injury Awareness Month		**OCT**	Occupational Therapy Month
JUNE 27	PTSD Awareness Day		**OCT**	Respiratory Therapy Week
AUG 17	World Pancreatic Cancer Day		**OC**	Critical Care Week
AUG 19	World Humanitarian Day		**NOV**	Nurse Practitioner Week

COMMON **ABBREVIATIONS** IN THE ICU

A C L S	Advanced Cardiac Life Support	L O C	Level of Consciousness
A N D	Allow Natural Death	M D	Medical Doctor
B M	Bowel Movement	M I	Myocardial Infarction
B P	Blood pressure	M R I	Magnetic Resonance Imaging
C B C	Complete blood count	M R P	Most Responsible Physician
C C O T	Critical Care Outreach Team	N A	Nurse's Aide
C P R	Cardiopulmonary Resuscitation	N G	Nasogastric Tube
C T	Computed Tomography	N P	Nurse Practitioner
C X R	Chest X-ray	N P O	Nothing by mouth
C V A	Cerebrovascular Accident	O G	Orogastric Tube
D N R	Do Not Resuscitate	O T	Occupational Therapist | Therapy
D V T	Deep Vein Thrombosis	P C A	Personal Care Aid
E C G | E K G	Electrocardiogram	P O	By mouth
E D	Emergency Department	P R N	As needed
E E G	Electroencephalogram	P S W	Personal Support Worker
E R	Emergency Room	P T	Physiotherapist | Physical Therapy
E T T	Endotracheal Tube	R N	Registered Nurse
G C S	Glasgow Coma Scale	R R	Respiratory Rate
G O C	Goals of Care	R T	Respiratory Therapist
H R	Heart rate	S L P	Speech Language Pathologist
I C U	Intensive Care Unit	S O B	Shortness of Breath
I P A C	Infection Prevention and Control	$S P O_2$	Blood Oxygen Saturation
I V	Intravenous	V S	Vital Signs

THE
JOURNAL

DISCLAIMER

The following Journal serves as an aid and a guide to facilitate note-taking. The Journal should not be relied upon to replace any advice from a qualified health professional, nor should it be understood to be a legal document. By using this Journal, you acknowledge that it is intended solely for personal use and is not a substitute for professional medical, legal, or other expert advice. Always consult a qualified professional regarding any health, legal, or other issues you may have. The Journal is not a legal document, nor should it be relied upon in legal proceedings, or seen as superior to any medical notes. You understand that respect and protection for patient privacy and confidentiality are of the utmost importance. Any notes taken within the Journal should be protected for the benefit of the patient. The creators and distributors of this Journal disclaim any liability for decisions made based on the information contained herein.

HOSPITAL CONTACT INFO

Before leaving the hospital after admission, gather this information.

HOSPITAL ADDRESS

EMAIL (IF APPLICABLE)

PHONE NUMBER(S)

FAX NUMBER(S)

HOSPITAL CONTACT INFO

VISITING HOURS

NURSE SHIFT CHANGE

ABOUT NURSING SHIFT CHANGE

Shift change is when patient transfer of care occurs between one staff nurse to another (e.g., day shift to night shift). During this time, important information regarding the patient's history, current status and care priorities are discussed. The chart, medications, intravenous infusions and specialty equipment are typically reviewed. Many ICUs limit visiting during shift change to respect patient privacy and limit interruptions that can lead to missed information exchanges.

VISITING INSTRUCTIONS / POLICY

WHAT HAPPENED ON
THE DAY OF **ADMISSION?**

THE STORY OF WHAT HAPPENED

....

....

....

....

....

....

....

....

....

....

....

....

....

....

....

....

....

....

....

....

HOSPITAL

FAMILY / FRIENDS PRESENT

EMERGENCY DEPARTMENT

ADMITTING PHYSICIAN

ADMITTING NURSE

ROOM

INTENSIVE CARE UNIT

ADMITTING PHYSICIAN

ADMITTING NURSE

ROOM

WHAT HAPPENED ON THE DAY OF **ADMISSION?**

DURING THE ADMISSION

- [ ] NOTIFY FAMILY
- [ ] NOTIFY FRIENDS
- [ ] NOTIFY EMPLOYER
- [ ] BRING PERSONAL BELONGINGS AND VALUABLES HOME

WHILE YOU WAIT FOR UPDATES

- [ ] REMEMBER TO EAT
- [ ] REMEMBER TO HYDRATE
- [ ] REMEMBER TO SLEEP
- [ ] REMEMBER TO TAKE BREAKS
- [ ] WRITE DOWN QUESTIONS

TESTS & PROCEDURES

- [ ] X-RAY
- [ ] ECG
- [ ] BLOODWORK
- [ ] CT SCAN
- [ ] BRONCHOSCOPY

- [ ] ADMISSION SWABS
- [ ] SUPPLEMENTAL OXYGEN
- [ ] INTUBATION
- [ ] IV INSERTION
- [ ] URINARY CATHETER

- [ ] FAMILY MEETING
- [ ] WOUND CARE
- [ ] SURGERY
- [ ] OTHER

NOTES

....

....

....

PROTIP: The first 12-24+ hours when a patient is admitted to an ICU is extremely busy for the care team. Wait until the patient's illness acuity has settled before asking the nursing staff to help fill in these details.

BEFORE YOU LEAVE THE ICU ON DAY 1

Ask the ward clerk for directions on how to call the unit for updates and when nursing shift change occurs.	Ask the ward clerk about visiting hours and the visiting policy (if applicable).	Have a trusted family member remove all valuables and jewelry from the patient and store at home.	Confirm the ICU team has the right contact information for the decision maker on file.

TODAY'S ENTRY IS COMPLETED BY: ....

THERAPEUTIC
JOURNAL

ICU PHYSICIAN: ....

TODAY'S DATE: ....

DAY NURSE: ....

ROOM #: ....

NIGHT NURSE: ....

NUMBER OF IV PUMPS

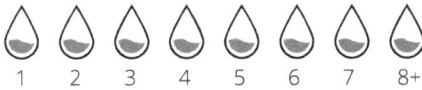

💧 💧 💧 💧 💧 💧 💧 💧
1   2   3   4   5   6   7   8+

IV LINES

☐ IV LINE   ☐ INTRAOSSEOUS
☐ CENTRAL LINE   ☐ PORT
☐ PICC LINE   ☐ OTHER
☐ DIALYSIS LINE

BREATHING SUPPORT

☐ INTUBATED   ☐ EXTUBATED
☐ VENTILATOR   ☐ HIGH FLOW
☐ TRACHEOSTOMY   ☐ NASAL PRONGS
☐ BIPAP / CPAP   ☐ ROOM AIR
☐ FACE MASK   ☐ OTHER

DAILY PROGRESS AND GOALS

LEVEL OF CONSCIOUSNESS

☐ AWAKE   ☐ SEIZURE
☐ ALERT   ☐ AGITATED
☐ ORIENTED   ☐ HALLUCINATIONS
☐ PARALYTIC MEDICATION   ☐ CONFUSED
☐ SEDATED   ☐ DELIRIOUS
☐ LETHARGIC   ☐ OTHER

NUTRITION

☐ NOTHING BY MOUTH   ☐ ICE CHIPS / CLEAR FLUIDS
☐ FEEDING TUBE   ☐ PUREED DIET
☐ FEEDS HELD   ☐ REGULAR
☐ TPN (IV)   ☐ OTHER

WOUNDS / INJURIES

....
....

EACH DAY, THERE MAY BE ONE OR MORE GOALS OF CARE THAT THE TEAM IS HOPING THE PATIENT WILL ACHIEVE.

....
....

NOTES

....
....
....

TESTS PERFORMED TODAY

- ☐ X-RAY
- ☐ CT SCAN
- ☐ MRI
- ☐ ULTRASOUND
- ☐ BLOOD TESTS
- ☐ BREATHING TRIAL
- ☐ SPUTUM / LUNG
- ☐ OTHER

INTERDISCIPLINARY ROUNDS

TODAY'S EXERCISES

- ☐ RANGE OF MOTION
- ☐ REPOSITIONING
- ☐ SIT AT BEDSIDE
- ☐ STAND AT BEDSIDE
- ☐ SIT IN CHAIR
- ☐ BICYCLE
- ☐ WALKING
- ☐ BEDREST

WHAT ARE THE MAJOR ISSUES / CONCERNS TODAY? IS THE PATIENT GETTING BETTER OR WORSE? WHAT ARE SHORT- & LONG-TERM GOALS?

TODAY YOU (PATIENT) FELT:

ANGRY TIRED SAD HAPPY EXCITED SEDATED

BECAUSE: ☐ OTHER

1.
2.
3.

TODAY I (CAREGIVER) FELT:

ANGRY TIRED SAD HAPPY EXCITED

BECAUSE: ☐ OTHER

1.
2.
3.

WHAT HAPPENED TODAY?

PATIENT EVENTS | NEWS | MAJOR WORLD EVENTS | FAMILY EVENTS | VISITORS | ACTIVITIES | ICU ENVIRONMENT | SOUNDS | LIFE UPDATES | HOLIDAYS | RECOVERY MILESTONE

TODAY WE ARE GRATEFUL FOR...

1.
2.
3.

TODAY'S MESSAGE OF HOPE

QUOTE OF THE DAY

"We are only as strong as we are united, as weak we are divided." - J.K. Rowling

THERAPEUTIC
JOURNAL

TODAY'S DATE: ....

ROOM #: ....

ICU PHYSICIAN: ....

DAY NURSE: ....

NIGHT NURSE: ....

NUMBER OF IV PUMPS

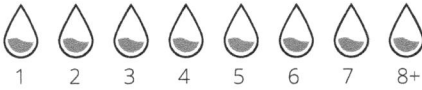

1   2   3   4   5   6   7   8+

IV LINES

- ☐ IV LINE
- ☐ CENTRAL LINE
- ☐ PICC LINE
- ☐ DIALYSIS LINE
- ☐ INTRAOSSEOUS
- ☐ PORT
- ☐ OTHER

BREATHING SUPPORT

- ☐ INTUBATED
- ☐ VENTILATOR
- ☐ TRACHEOSTOMY
- ☐ BIPAP / CPAP
- ☐ FACE MASK
- ☐ EXTUBATED
- ☐ HIGH FLOW
- ☐ NASAL PRONGS
- ☐ ROOM AIR
- ☐ OTHER

LEVEL OF CONSCIOUSNESS

- ☐ AWAKE
- ☐ ALERT
- ☐ ORIENTED
- ☐ PARALYTIC MEDICATION
- ☐ SEDATED
- ☐ LETHARGIC
- ☐ SEIZURE
- ☐ AGITATED
- ☐ HALLUCINATIONS
- ☐ CONFUSED
- ☐ DELIRIOUS
- ☐ OTHER

NUTRITION

- ☐ NOTHING BY MOUTH
- ☐ FEEDING TUBE
- ☐ FEEDS HELD
- ☐ TPN (IV)
- ☐ ICE CHIPS / CLEAR FLUIDS
- ☐ PUREED DIET
- ☐ REGULAR
- ☐ OTHER

WOUNDS / INJURIES

....

....

DAILY PROGRESS AND GOALS

EACH DAY, THERE MAY BE ONE OR MORE GOALS OF CARE THAT THE TEAM IS HOPING THE PATIENT WILL ACHIEVE.

....

....

NOTES

....

....

....

TESTS PERFORMED TODAY

- ☐ X-RAY
- ☐ CT SCAN
- ☐ MRI
- ☐ ULTRASOUND
- ☐ BLOOD TESTS
- ☐ BREATHING TRIAL
- ☐ SPUTUM / LUNG
- ☐ OTHER

TODAY'S EXERCISES

- ☐ RANGE OF MOTION
- ☐ REPOSITIONING
- ☐ SIT AT BEDSIDE
- ☐ STAND AT BEDSIDE
- ☐ SIT IN CHAIR
- ☐ BICYCLE
- ☐ WALKING
- ☐ BEDREST

INTERDISCIPLINARY ROUNDS

WHAT ARE THE MAJOR ISSUES / CONCERNS TODAY? IS THE PATIENT GETTING BETTER OR WORSE? WHAT ARE SHORT- & LONG-TERM GOALS?

TODAY YOU (PATIENT) FELT:

ANGRY   TIRED   SAD   HAPPY   EXCITED   SEDATED

BECAUSE: ☐ OTHER

1.
2.
3.

TODAY I (CAREGIVER) FELT:

ANGRY   TIRED   SAD   HAPPY   EXCITED

BECAUSE: ☐ OTHER

1.
2.
3.

WHAT HAPPENED TODAY?

PATIENT EVENTS | NEWS | MAJOR WORLD EVENTS | FAMILY EVENTS | VISITORS | ACTIVITIES | ICU ENVIRONMENT | SOUNDS | LIFE UPDATES | HOLIDAYS | RECOVERY MILESTONE

TODAY WE ARE GRATEFUL FOR...

1.
2.
3.

TODAY'S MESSAGE OF HOPE

QUOTE OF THE DAY

"We grieve because we love. The intensity of the grief often proclaims the depth of our love." - Gary Roe

TODAY'S ENTRY IS COMPLETED BY: ....

THERAPEUTIC
JOURNAL

TODAY'S DATE: ....

ROOM #: ....

ICU PHYSICIAN: ....

DAY NURSE: ....

NIGHT NURSE: ....

NUMBER OF IV PUMPS

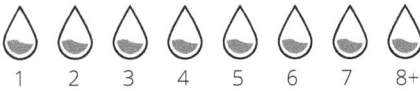

1   2   3   4   5   6   7   8+

IV LINES

- [ ] IV LINE
- [ ] CENTRAL LINE
- [ ] PICC LINE
- [ ] DIALYSIS LINE
- [ ] INTRAOSSEOUS
- [ ] PORT
- [ ] OTHER

BREATHING SUPPORT

- [ ] INTUBATED
- [ ] VENTILATOR
- [ ] TRACHEOSTOMY
- [ ] BIPAP / CPAP
- [ ] FACE MASK
- [ ] EXTUBATED
- [ ] HIGH FLOW
- [ ] NASAL PRONGS
- [ ] ROOM AIR
- [ ] OTHER

LEVEL OF CONSCIOUSNESS

- [ ] AWAKE
- [ ] ALERT
- [ ] ORIENTED
- [ ] PARALYTIC MEDICATION
- [ ] SEDATED
- [ ] LETHARGIC
- [ ] SEIZURE
- [ ] AGITATED
- [ ] HALLUCINATIONS
- [ ] CONFUSED
- [ ] DELIRIOUS
- [ ] OTHER

NUTRITION

- [ ] NOTHING BY MOUTH
- [ ] FEEDING TUBE
- [ ] FEEDS HELD
- [ ] TPN (IV)
- [ ] ICE CHIPS / CLEAR FLUIDS
- [ ] PUREED DIET
- [ ] REGULAR
- [ ] OTHER

WOUNDS / INJURIES

....

....

DAILY PROGRESS AND GOALS

EACH DAY, THERE MAY BE ONE OR MORE GOALS OF CARE THAT THE TEAM IS HOPING THE PATIENT WILL ACHIEVE.

....

....

NOTES

....

....

....

....

TESTS PERFORMED TODAY

☐ X-RAY　　　　☐ BLOOD TESTS

☐ CT SCAN　　　☐ BREATHING TRIAL

☐ MRI　　　　　☐ SPUTUM / LUNG

☐ ULTRASOUND　☐ OTHER

INTERDISCIPLINARY ROUNDS

TODAY'S EXERCISES

☐ RANGE OF MOTION　☐ SIT IN CHAIR

☐ REPOSITIONING　　☐ BICYCLE

☐ SIT AT BEDSIDE　　☐ WALKING

☐ STAND AT BEDSIDE　☐ BEDREST

WHAT ARE THE MAJOR ISSUES / CONCERNS TODAY? IS THE PATIENT GETTING BETTER OR WORSE? WHAT ARE SHORT- & LONG-TERM GOALS?

....

....

....

....

TODAY YOU (PATIENT) FELT:

😠　😫　🙁　🙂　😆　😴
ANGRY　TIRED　SAD　HAPPY　EXCITED　SEDATED

BECAUSE:　　　　　☐ OTHER
1. ....
2. ....
3. ....

TODAY I (CAREGIVER) FELT:

😠　😫　🙁　🙂　😆
ANGRY　TIRED　SAD　HAPPY　EXCITED

BECAUSE:　　　　　☐ OTHER
1. ....
2. ....
3. ....

WHAT HAPPENED TODAY?

PATIENT EVENTS | NEWS | MAJOR WORLD EVENTS | FAMILY EVENTS | VISITORS | ACTIVITIES | ICU ENVIRONMENT | SOUNDS | LIFE UPDATES | HOLIDAYS | RECOVERY MILESTONE

....

....

....

....

....

....

....

TODAY WE ARE GRATEFUL FOR...

1. ....

2. ....

3. ....

TODAY'S MESSAGE OF HOPE

....

....

....

QUOTE OF THE DAY

"Remember, tough times don't last, but tough people do." - Unknown

THERAPEUTIC
JOURNAL

TODAY'S DATE: ....

ROOM #: ....

ICU PHYSICIAN: ....

DAY NURSE: ....

NIGHT NURSE: ....

NUMBER OF IV PUMPS

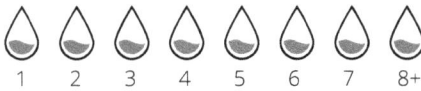

1 2 3 4 5 6 7 8+

IV LINES

☐ IV LINE   ☐ INTRAOSSEOUS
☐ CENTRAL LINE   ☐ PORT
☐ PICC LINE   ☐ OTHER
☐ DIALYSIS LINE

BREATHING SUPPORT

☐ INTUBATED   ☐ EXTUBATED
☐ VENTILATOR   ☐ HIGH FLOW
☐ TRACHEOSTOMY   ☐ NASAL PRONGS
☐ BIPAP / CPAP   ☐ ROOM AIR
☐ FACE MASK   ☐ OTHER

LEVEL OF CONSCIOUSNESS

☐ AWAKE   ☐ SEIZURE
☐ ALERT   ☐ AGITATED
☐ ORIENTED   ☐ HALLUCINATIONS
☐ PARALYTIC MEDICATION   ☐ CONFUSED
☐ SEDATED   ☐ DELIRIOUS
☐ LETHARGIC   ☐ OTHER

NUTRITION

☐ NOTHING BY MOUTH   ☐ ICE CHIPS / CLEAR FLUIDS
☐ FEEDING TUBE   ☐ PUREED DIET
☐ FEEDS HELD   ☐ REGULAR
☐ TPN (IV)   ☐ OTHER

WOUNDS / INJURIES

....
....

DAILY PROGRESS AND GOALS

EACH DAY, THERE MAY BE ONE OR MORE GOALS OF CARE THAT THE TEAM IS HOPING THE PATIENT WILL ACHIEVE.

....
....

NOTES

....
....
....

TESTS PERFORMED TODAY

☐ X-RAY   ☐ BLOOD TESTS

☐ CT SCAN   ☐ BREATHING TRIAL

☐ MRI   ☐ SPUTUM / LUNG

☐ ULTRASOUND   ☐ OTHER

INTERDISCIPLINARY ROUNDS

TODAY'S EXERCISES

☐ RANGE OF MOTION   ☐ SIT IN CHAIR

☐ REPOSITIONING   ☐ BICYCLE

☐ SIT AT BEDSIDE   ☐ WALKING

☐ STAND AT BEDSIDE   ☐ BEDREST

WHAT ARE THE MAJOR ISSUES / CONCERNS TODAY? IS THE PATIENT GETTING BETTER OR WORSE? WHAT ARE SHORT- & LONG-TERM GOALS?

TODAY YOU (PATIENT) FELT:

ANGRY   TIRED   SAD   HAPPY   EXCITED   SEDATED

BECAUSE: ☐ OTHER

1.

2.

3.

TODAY I (CAREGIVER) FELT:

ANGRY   TIRED   SAD   HAPPY   EXCITED

BECAUSE: ☐ OTHER

1.

2.

3.

WHAT HAPPENED TODAY?

PATIENT EVENTS | NEWS | MAJOR WORLD EVENTS | FAMILY EVENTS | VISITORS | ACTIVITIES | ICU ENVIRONMENT | SOUNDS | LIFE UPDATES | HOLIDAYS | RECOVERY MILESTONE

TODAY WE ARE GRATEFUL FOR...

1.

2.

3.

TODAY'S MESSAGE OF HOPE

QUOTE OF THE DAY

"Medicine works to cure your body. Our friendship works to cure your soul." - Euripides

TODAY'S ENTRY IS COMPLETED BY: ....

THERAPEUTIC
JOURNAL

TODAY'S DATE: ....

ROOM #: ....

ICU PHYSICIAN: ....

DAY NURSE: ....

NIGHT NURSE: ....

NUMBER OF IV PUMPS

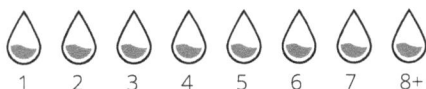

1   2   3   4   5   6   7   8+

IV LINES

- ☐ IV LINE
- ☐ CENTRAL LINE
- ☐ PICC LINE
- ☐ DIALYSIS LINE
- ☐ INTRAOSSEOUS
- ☐ PORT
- ☐ OTHER

BREATHING SUPPORT

- ☐ INTUBATED
- ☐ VENTILATOR
- ☐ TRACHEOSTOMY
- ☐ BIPAP / CPAP
- ☐ FACE MASK
- ☐ EXTUBATED
- ☐ HIGH FLOW
- ☐ NASAL PRONGS
- ☐ ROOM AIR
- ☐ OTHER

LEVEL OF CONSCIOUSNESS

- ☐ AWAKE
- ☐ ALERT
- ☐ ORIENTED
- ☐ PARALYTIC MEDICATION
- ☐ SEDATED
- ☐ LETHARGIC
- ☐ SEIZURE
- ☐ AGITATED
- ☐ HALLUCINATIONS
- ☐ CONFUSED
- ☐ DELIRIOUS
- ☐ OTHER

NUTRITION

- ☐ NOTHING BY MOUTH
- ☐ FEEDING TUBE
- ☐ FEEDS HELD
- ☐ TPN (IV)
- ☐ ICE CHIPS / CLEAR FLUIDS
- ☐ PUREED DIET
- ☐ REGULAR
- ☐ OTHER

WOUNDS / INJURIES

....

....

DAILY PROGRESS AND GOALS

EACH DAY, THERE MAY BE ONE OR MORE GOALS OF CARE THAT THE TEAM IS HOPING THE PATIENT WILL ACHIEVE.

....

....

NOTES

....

....

....

TESTS PERFORMED TODAY

☐ X-RAY   ☐ BLOOD TESTS

☐ CT SCAN   ☐ BREATHING TRIAL

☐ MRI   ☐ SPUTUM / LUNG

☐ ULTRASOUND   ☐ OTHER

INTERDISCIPLINARY ROUNDS

TODAY'S EXERCISES

☐ RANGE OF MOTION   ☐ SIT IN CHAIR

☐ REPOSITIONING   ☐ BICYCLE

☐ SIT AT BEDSIDE   ☐ WALKING

☐ STAND AT BEDSIDE   ☐ BEDREST

WHAT ARE THE MAJOR ISSUES / CONCERNS TODAY? IS THE PATIENT GETTING BETTER OR WORSE? WHAT ARE SHORT- & LONG-TERM GOALS?

....

....

....

....

TODAY YOU (PATIENT) FELT:

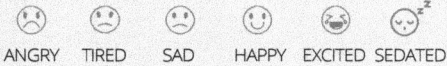

😠   😩   🙁   🙂   😆   😴
ANGRY   TIRED   SAD   HAPPY   EXCITED SEDATED

BECAUSE: ☐ OTHER

1. ....

2. ....

3. ....

TODAY I (CAREGIVER) FELT:

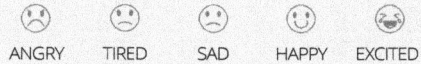

😠   😩   🙁   🙂   😆
ANGRY   TIRED   SAD   HAPPY   EXCITED

BECAUSE: ☐ OTHER

1. ....

2. ....

3. ....

WHAT HAPPENED TODAY?

PATIENT EVENTS | NEWS | MAJOR WORLD EVENTS | FAMILY EVENTS | VISITORS | ACTIVITIES | ICU ENVIRONMENT | SOUNDS | LIFE UPDATES | HOLIDAYS | RECOVERY MILESTONE

....

....

....

....

....

....

TODAY WE ARE GRATEFUL FOR...

1. ....

2. ....

3. ....

TODAY'S MESSAGE OF HOPE

....

....

....

....

QUOTE OF THE DAY

"Better is possible. It does not take genius. It takes diligence. It takes moral clarity. It takes ingenuity. And above all, it takes a willingness to try." - Atul Gawande

TODAY'S ENTRY IS COMPLETED BY: ....

THERAPEUTIC
JOURNAL

TODAY'S DATE: ....

ROOM #: ....

ICU PHYSICIAN: ....

DAY NURSE: ....

NIGHT NURSE: ....

NUMBER OF IV PUMPS

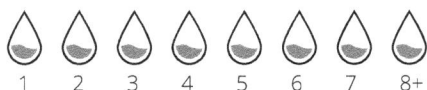

◊ ◊ ◊ ◊ ◊ ◊ ◊ ◊
1   2   3   4   5   6   7   8+

IV LINES

☐ IV LINE   ☐ INTRAOSSEOUS
☐ CENTRAL LINE   ☐ PORT
☐ PICC LINE   ☐ OTHER
☐ DIALYSIS LINE

BREATHING SUPPORT

☐ INTUBATED   ☐ EXTUBATED
☐ VENTILATOR   ☐ HIGH FLOW
☐ TRACHEOSTOMY   ☐ NASAL PRONGS
☐ BIPAP / CPAP   ☐ ROOM AIR
☐ FACE MASK   ☐ OTHER

LEVEL OF CONSCIOUSNESS

☐ AWAKE   ☐ SEIZURE
☐ ALERT   ☐ AGITATED
☐ ORIENTED   ☐ HALLUCINATIONS
☐ PARALYTIC MEDICATION   ☐ CONFUSED
☐ SEDATED   ☐ DELIRIOUS
☐ LETHARGIC   ☐ OTHER

NUTRITION

☐ NOTHING BY MOUTH   ☐ ICE CHIPS / CLEAR FLUIDS
☐ FEEDING TUBE   ☐ PUREED DIET
☐ FEEDS HELD   ☐ REGULAR
☐ TPN (IV)   ☐ OTHER

WOUNDS / INJURIES

....

....

DAILY PROGRESS AND GOALS

EACH DAY, THERE MAY BE ONE OR MORE GOALS OF CARE THAT THE TEAM IS HOPING THE PATIENT WILL ACHIEVE.

....

....

NOTES

....

....

....

TESTS PERFORMED TODAY

☐ X-RAY   ☐ BLOOD TESTS

☐ CT SCAN   ☐ BREATHING TRIAL

☐ MRI   ☐ SPUTUM / LUNG

☐ ULTRASOUND   ☐ OTHER

INTERDISCIPLINARY ROUNDS

TODAY'S EXERCISES

☐ RANGE OF MOTION   ☐ SIT IN CHAIR

☐ REPOSITIONING   ☐ BICYCLE

☐ SIT AT BEDSIDE   ☐ WALKING

☐ STAND AT BEDSIDE   ☐ BEDREST

WHAT ARE THE MAJOR ISSUES / CONCERNS TODAY? IS THE PATIENT GETTING BETTER OR WORSE? WHAT ARE SHORT- & LONG-TERM GOALS?

TODAY YOU (PATIENT) FELT:

ANGRY   TIRED   SAD   HAPPY   EXCITED   SEDATED

BECAUSE: ☐ OTHER

1.

2.

3.

TODAY I (CAREGIVER) FELT:

ANGRY   TIRED   SAD   HAPPY   EXCITED

BECAUSE: ☐ OTHER

1.

2.

3.

WHAT HAPPENED TODAY?

PATIENT EVENTS | NEWS | MAJOR WORLD EVENTS | FAMILY EVENTS | VISITORS | ACTIVITIES | ICU ENVIRONMENT | SOUNDS | LIFE UPDATES | HOLIDAYS | RECOVERY MILESTONE

TODAY WE ARE GRATEFUL FOR...

1.

2.

3.

TODAY'S MESSAGE OF HOPE

QUOTE OF THE DAY

"Courage is not having the strength to go on, it is going on when you don't have the strength." - Theodore Roosevelt

53

THERAPEUTIC
JOURNAL

TODAY'S DATE: ....

ROOM #: ....

ICU PHYSICIAN: ....

DAY NURSE: ....

NIGHT NURSE: ....

NUMBER OF IV PUMPS

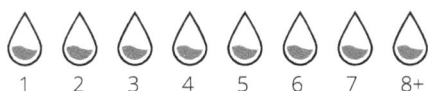

1 2 3 4 5 6 7 8+

IV LINES

- ☐ IV LINE
- ☐ CENTRAL LINE
- ☐ PICC LINE
- ☐ DIALYSIS LINE
- ☐ INTRAOSSEOUS
- ☐ PORT
- ☐ OTHER

BREATHING SUPPORT

- ☐ INTUBATED
- ☐ VENTILATOR
- ☐ TRACHEOSTOMY
- ☐ BIPAP / CPAP
- ☐ FACE MASK
- ☐ EXTUBATED
- ☐ HIGH FLOW
- ☐ NASAL PRONGS
- ☐ ROOM AIR
- ☐ OTHER

LEVEL OF CONSCIOUSNESS

- ☐ AWAKE
- ☐ ALERT
- ☐ ORIENTED
- ☐ PARALYTIC MEDICATION
- ☐ SEDATED
- ☐ LETHARGIC
- ☐ SEIZURE
- ☐ AGITATED
- ☐ HALLUCINATIONS
- ☐ CONFUSED
- ☐ DELIRIOUS
- ☐ OTHER

NUTRITION

- ☐ NOTHING BY MOUTH
- ☐ FEEDING TUBE
- ☐ FEEDS HELD
- ☐ TPN (IV)
- ☐ ICE CHIPS / CLEAR FLUIDS
- ☐ PUREED DIET
- ☐ REGULAR
- ☐ OTHER

WOUNDS / INJURIES

....

....

DAILY PROGRESS AND GOALS

EACH DAY, THERE MAY BE ONE OR MORE GOALS OF CARE THAT THE TEAM IS HOPING THE PATIENT WILL ACHIEVE.

....

....

NOTES

....

....

....

TESTS PERFORMED TODAY

- [ ] X-RAY
- [ ] CT SCAN
- [ ] MRI
- [ ] ULTRASOUND
- [ ] BLOOD TESTS
- [ ] BREATHING TRIAL
- [ ] SPUTUM / LUNG
- [ ] OTHER

TODAY'S EXERCISES

- [ ] RANGE OF MOTION
- [ ] REPOSITIONING
- [ ] SIT AT BEDSIDE
- [ ] STAND AT BEDSIDE
- [ ] SIT IN CHAIR
- [ ] BICYCLE
- [ ] WALKING
- [ ] BEDREST

INTERDISCIPLINARY ROUNDS

WHAT ARE THE MAJOR ISSUES / CONCERNS TODAY? IS THE PATIENT GETTING BETTER OR WORSE? WHAT ARE SHORT- & LONG-TERM GOALS?

TODAY YOU (PATIENT) FELT:

ANGRY   TIRED   SAD   HAPPY   EXCITED   SEDATED

BECAUSE: [ ] OTHER

1.
2.
3.

TODAY I (CAREGIVER) FELT:

ANGRY   TIRED   SAD   HAPPY   EXCITED

BECAUSE: [ ] OTHER

1.
2.
3.

WHAT HAPPENED TODAY?

PATIENT EVENTS | NEWS | MAJOR WORLD EVENTS | FAMILY EVENTS | VISITORS | ACTIVITIES | ICU ENVIRONMENT | SOUNDS | LIFE UPDATES | HOLIDAYS | RECOVERY MILESTONE

TODAY WE ARE GRATEFUL FOR...

1.
2.
3.

TODAY'S MESSAGE OF HOPE

QUOTE OF THE DAY

"Life doesn't get easier or more forgiving, we get stronger and more resilient." - Steve Maraboli

TODAY'S ENTRY IS COMPLETED BY: ....

THERAPEUTIC
JOURNAL

TODAY'S DATE: ....

ROOM #: ....

ICU PHYSICIAN: ....

DAY NURSE: ....

NIGHT NURSE: ....

NUMBER OF IV PUMPS

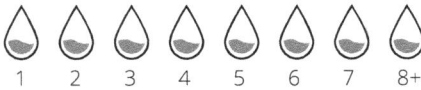

1   2   3   4   5   6   7   8+

IV LINES

- [ ] IV LINE
- [ ] CENTRAL LINE
- [ ] PICC LINE
- [ ] DIALYSIS LINE
- [ ] INTRAOSSEOUS
- [ ] PORT
- [ ] OTHER

BREATHING SUPPORT

- [ ] INTUBATED
- [ ] VENTILATOR
- [ ] TRACHEOSTOMY
- [ ] BIPAP / CPAP
- [ ] FACE MASK
- [ ] EXTUBATED
- [ ] HIGH FLOW
- [ ] NASAL PRONGS
- [ ] ROOM AIR
- [ ] OTHER

LEVEL OF CONSCIOUSNESS

- [ ] AWAKE
- [ ] ALERT
- [ ] ORIENTED
- [ ] PARALYTIC MEDICATION
- [ ] SEDATED
- [ ] LETHARGIC
- [ ] SEIZURE
- [ ] AGITATED
- [ ] HALLUCINATIONS
- [ ] CONFUSED
- [ ] DELIRIOUS
- [ ] OTHER

NUTRITION

- [ ] NOTHING BY MOUTH
- [ ] FEEDING TUBE
- [ ] FEEDS HELD
- [ ] TPN (IV)
- [ ] ICE CHIPS / CLEAR FLUIDS
- [ ] PUREED DIET
- [ ] REGULAR
- [ ] OTHER

WOUNDS / INJURIES

DAILY PROGRESS AND GOALS

EACH DAY, THERE MAY BE ONE OR MORE GOALS OF CARE THAT THE TEAM IS HOPING THE PATIENT WILL ACHIEVE.

NOTES

TESTS PERFORMED TODAY

☐ X-RAY   ☐ BLOOD TESTS

☐ CT SCAN   ☐ BREATHING TRIAL

☐ MRI   ☐ SPUTUM / LUNG

☐ ULTRASOUND   ☐ OTHER

TODAY'S EXERCISES

☐ RANGE OF MOTION   ☐ SIT IN CHAIR

☐ REPOSITIONING   ☐ BICYCLE

☐ SIT AT BEDSIDE   ☐ WALKING

☐ STAND AT BEDSIDE   ☐ BEDREST

INTERDISCIPLINARY ROUNDS

WHAT ARE THE MAJOR ISSUES / CONCERNS TODAY? IS THE PATIENT GETTING BETTER OR WORSE? WHAT ARE SHORT- & LONG-TERM GOALS?

....

....

....

TODAY YOU (PATIENT) FELT:

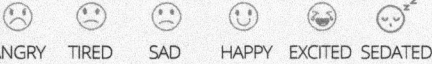

ANGRY   TIRED   SAD   HAPPY   EXCITED   SEDATED

BECAUSE: ☐ OTHER

1. ....

2. ....

3. ....

TODAY I (CAREGIVER) FELT:

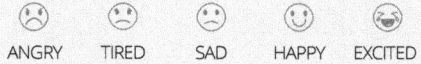

ANGRY   TIRED   SAD   HAPPY   EXCITED

BECAUSE: ☐ OTHER

1. ....

2. ....

3. ....

WHAT HAPPENED TODAY?

PATIENT EVENTS | NEWS | MAJOR WORLD EVENTS | FAMILY EVENTS | VISITORS | ACTIVITIES | ICU ENVIRONMENT | SOUNDS | LIFE UPDATES | HOLIDAYS | RECOVERY MILESTONE

....

....

....

....

....

TODAY WE ARE GRATEFUL FOR...

1. ....

2. ....

3. ....

TODAY'S MESSAGE OF HOPE

....

....

....

QUOTE OF THE DAY

"Where there is no struggle, there is no strength."
- Oprah Winfrey

TODAY'S ENTRY IS COMPLETED BY: ....

THERAPEUTIC
JOURNAL

TODAY'S DATE: ....

ROOM #: ....

ICU PHYSICIAN: ....

DAY NURSE: ....

NIGHT NURSE: ....

NUMBER OF IV PUMPS

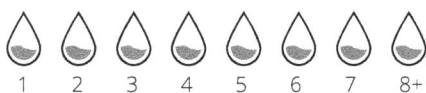

💧 💧 💧 💧 💧 💧 💧 💧
1   2   3   4   5   6   7   8+

IV LINES

☐ IV LINE   ☐ INTRAOSSEOUS

☐ CENTRAL LINE   ☐ PORT

☐ PICC LINE   ☐ OTHER

☐ DIALYSIS LINE

BREATHING SUPPORT

☐ INTUBATED   ☐ EXTUBATED

☐ VENTILATOR   ☐ HIGH FLOW

☐ TRACHEOSTOMY   ☐ NASAL PRONGS

☐ BIPAP / CPAP   ☐ ROOM AIR

☐ FACE MASK   ☐ OTHER

LEVEL OF CONSCIOUSNESS

☐ AWAKE   ☐ SEIZURE

☐ ALERT   ☐ AGITATED

☐ ORIENTED   ☐ HALLUCINATIONS

☐ PARALYTIC MEDICATION   ☐ CONFUSED

☐ SEDATED   ☐ DELIRIOUS

☐ LETHARGIC   ☐ OTHER

NUTRITION

☐ NOTHING BY MOUTH   ☐ ICE CHIPS / CLEAR FLUIDS

☐ FEEDING TUBE   ☐ PUREED DIET

☐ FEEDS HELD   ☐ REGULAR

☐ TPN (IV)   ☐ OTHER

WOUNDS / INJURIES

....

....

DAILY PROGRESS AND GOALS

EACH DAY, THERE MAY BE ONE OR MORE GOALS OF CARE THAT THE TEAM IS HOPING THE PATIENT WILL ACHIEVE.

....

....

NOTES

....

....

....

TESTS PERFORMED TODAY

- ☐ X-RAY
- ☐ CT SCAN
- ☐ MRI
- ☐ ULTRASOUND
- ☐ BLOOD TESTS
- ☐ BREATHING TRIAL
- ☐ SPUTUM / LUNG
- ☐ OTHER

INTERDISCIPLINARY ROUNDS

TODAY'S EXERCISES

- ☐ RANGE OF MOTION
- ☐ REPOSITIONING
- ☐ SIT AT BEDSIDE
- ☐ STAND AT BEDSIDE
- ☐ SIT IN CHAIR
- ☐ BICYCLE
- ☐ WALKING
- ☐ BEDREST

WHAT ARE THE MAJOR ISSUES / CONCERNS TODAY? IS THE PATIENT GETTING BETTER OR WORSE? WHAT ARE SHORT- & LONG-TERM GOALS?

TODAY YOU (PATIENT) FELT:

ANGRY   TIRED   SAD   HAPPY   EXCITED   SEDATED

BECAUSE:
☐ OTHER
1.
2.
3.

TODAY I (CAREGIVER) FELT:

ANGRY   TIRED   SAD   HAPPY   EXCITED

BECAUSE:
☐ OTHER
1.
2.
3.

WHAT HAPPENED TODAY?

PATIENT EVENTS | NEWS | MAJOR WORLD EVENTS | FAMILY EVENTS | VISITORS | ACTIVITIES | ICU ENVIRONMENT | SOUNDS | LIFE UPDATES | HOLIDAYS | RECOVERY MILESTONE

TODAY WE ARE GRATEFUL FOR...

1.
2.
3.

TODAY'S MESSAGE OF HOPE

QUOTE OF THE DAY

"A hero is an ordinary individual who finds the strength to persevere and endure in spite of overwhelming obstacles."
- Christopher Reeve

THERAPEUTIC
JOURNAL

TODAY'S DATE: ....

ROOM #: ....

ICU PHYSICIAN: ....

DAY NURSE: ....

NIGHT NURSE: ....

NUMBER OF IV PUMPS

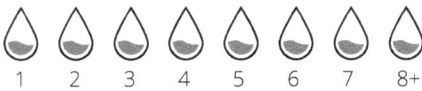

1   2   3   4   5   6   7   8+

IV LINES

- ☐ IV LINE
- ☐ CENTRAL LINE
- ☐ PICC LINE
- ☐ DIALYSIS LINE
- ☐ INTRAOSSEOUS
- ☐ PORT
- ☐ OTHER

BREATHING SUPPORT

- ☐ INTUBATED
- ☐ VENTILATOR
- ☐ TRACHEOSTOMY
- ☐ BIPAP / CPAP
- ☐ FACE MASK
- ☐ EXTUBATED
- ☐ HIGH FLOW
- ☐ NASAL PRONGS
- ☐ ROOM AIR
- ☐ OTHER

DAILY PROGRESS AND GOALS

LEVEL OF CONSCIOUSNESS

- ☐ AWAKE
- ☐ ALERT
- ☐ ORIENTED
- ☐ PARALYTIC MEDICATION
- ☐ SEDATED
- ☐ LETHARGIC
- ☐ SEIZURE
- ☐ AGITATED
- ☐ HALLUCINATIONS
- ☐ CONFUSED
- ☐ DELIRIOUS
- ☐ OTHER

NUTRITION

- ☐ NOTHING BY MOUTH
- ☐ FEEDING TUBE
- ☐ FEEDS HELD
- ☐ TPN (IV)
- ☐ ICE CHIPS / CLEAR FLUIDS
- ☐ PUREED DIET
- ☐ REGULAR
- ☐ OTHER

WOUNDS / INJURIES

EACH DAY, THERE MAY BE ONE OR MORE GOALS OF CARE THAT THE TEAM IS HOPING THE PATIENT WILL ACHIEVE.

NOTES

TESTS PERFORMED TODAY

- ☐ X-RAY
- ☐ CT SCAN
- ☐ MRI
- ☐ ULTRASOUND

- ☐ BLOOD TESTS
- ☐ BREATHING TRIAL
- ☐ SPUTUM / LUNG
- ☐ OTHER

TODAY'S EXERCISES

- ☐ RANGE OF MOTION
- ☐ REPOSITIONING
- ☐ SIT AT BEDSIDE
- ☐ STAND AT BEDSIDE

- ☐ SIT IN CHAIR
- ☐ BICYCLE
- ☐ WALKING
- ☐ BEDREST

INTERDISCIPLINARY ROUNDS

WHAT ARE THE MAJOR ISSUES / CONCERNS TODAY? IS THE PATIENT GETTING BETTER OR WORSE? WHAT ARE SHORT- & LONG-TERM GOALS?

TODAY YOU (PATIENT) FELT:

ANGRY TIRED SAD HAPPY EXCITED SEDATED

BECAUSE:
☐ OTHER
1.
2.
3.

TODAY I (CAREGIVER) FELT:

ANGRY TIRED SAD HAPPY EXCITED

BECAUSE:
☐ OTHER
1.
2.
3.

WHAT HAPPENED TODAY?

PATIENT EVENTS | NEWS | MAJOR WORLD EVENTS | FAMILY EVENTS | VISITORS | ACTIVITIES | ICU ENVIRONMENT | SOUNDS | LIFE UPDATES | HOLIDAYS | RECOVERY MILESTONE

TODAY WE ARE GRATEFUL FOR...

1.
2.
3.

TODAY'S MESSAGE OF HOPE

QUOTE OF THE DAY

"Hope is the only thing stronger than fear." - Unknown

TODAY'S ENTRY IS COMPLETED BY: ....

THERAPEUTIC
JOURNAL

TODAY'S DATE: ....

ROOM #: ....

ICU PHYSICIAN: ....

DAY NURSE: ....

NIGHT NURSE: ....

NUMBER OF IV PUMPS

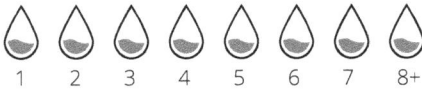

1 2 3 4 5 6 7 8+

IV LINES

- ☐ IV LINE
- ☐ CENTRAL LINE
- ☐ PICC LINE
- ☐ DIALYSIS LINE
- ☐ INTRAOSSEOUS
- ☐ PORT
- ☐ OTHER

BREATHING SUPPORT

- ☐ INTUBATED
- ☐ VENTILATOR
- ☐ TRACHEOSTOMY
- ☐ BIPAP / CPAP
- ☐ FACE MASK
- ☐ EXTUBATED
- ☐ HIGH FLOW
- ☐ NASAL PRONGS
- ☐ ROOM AIR
- ☐ OTHER

LEVEL OF CONSCIOUSNESS

- ☐ AWAKE
- ☐ ALERT
- ☐ ORIENTED
- ☐ PARALYTIC MEDICATION
- ☐ SEDATED
- ☐ LETHARGIC
- ☐ SEIZURE
- ☐ AGITATED
- ☐ HALLUCINATIONS
- ☐ CONFUSED
- ☐ DELIRIOUS
- ☐ OTHER

NUTRITION

- ☐ NOTHING BY MOUTH
- ☐ FEEDING TUBE
- ☐ FEEDS HELD
- ☐ TPN (IV)
- ☐ ICE CHIPS / CLEAR FLUIDS
- ☐ PUREED DIET
- ☐ REGULAR
- ☐ OTHER

WOUNDS / INJURIES

....
....

DAILY PROGRESS AND GOALS

EACH DAY, THERE MAY BE ONE OR MORE GOALS OF CARE THAT THE TEAM IS HOPING THE PATIENT WILL ACHIEVE.

....
....

NOTES

....
....
....

TESTS PERFORMED TODAY

☐ X-RAY ☐ BLOOD TESTS

☐ CT SCAN ☐ BREATHING TRIAL

☐ MRI ☐ SPUTUM / LUNG

☐ ULTRASOUND ☐ OTHER

INTERDISCIPLINARY ROUNDS

TODAY'S EXERCISES

☐ RANGE OF MOTION ☐ SIT IN CHAIR

☐ REPOSITIONING ☐ BICYCLE

☐ SIT AT BEDSIDE ☐ WALKING

☐ STAND AT BEDSIDE ☐ BEDREST

WHAT ARE THE MAJOR ISSUES / CONCERNS TODAY? IS THE PATIENT GETTING BETTER OR WORSE? WHAT ARE SHORT- & LONG-TERM GOALS?

TODAY YOU (PATIENT) FELT:

😠 😒 🙁 🙂 😄 😴
ANGRY TIRED SAD HAPPY EXCITED SEDATED

BECAUSE: ☐ OTHER

1. _____

2. _____

3. _____

TODAY I (CAREGIVER) FELT:

😠 😒 🙁 🙂 😄
ANGRY TIRED SAD HAPPY EXCITED

BECAUSE: ☐ OTHER

1. _____

2. _____

3. _____

WHAT HAPPENED TODAY?

PATIENT EVENTS | NEWS | MAJOR WORLD EVENTS | FAMILY EVENTS | VISITORS | ACTIVITIES | ICU ENVIRONMENT | SOUNDS | LIFE UPDATES | HOLIDAYS | RECOVERY MILESTONE

TODAY WE ARE GRATEFUL FOR...

1. _____

2. _____

3. _____

TODAY'S MESSAGE OF HOPE

QUOTE OF THE DAY

"When something bad happens, you have three choices: You can either let it define you, let it destroy you or let it strengthen you." - Unknown

63

TODAY'S ENTRY IS COMPLETED BY: ....

THERAPEUTIC
JOURNAL

TODAY'S DATE: ....

ROOM #: ....

ICU PHYSICIAN: ....

DAY NURSE: ....

NIGHT NURSE: ....

NUMBER OF IV PUMPS

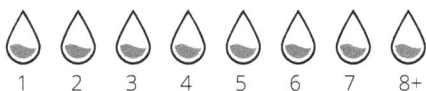

1   2   3   4   5   6   7   8+

IV LINES

- [ ] IV LINE
- [ ] CENTRAL LINE
- [ ] PICC LINE
- [ ] DIALYSIS LINE
- [ ] INTRAOSSEOUS
- [ ] PORT
- [ ] OTHER

BREATHING SUPPORT

- [ ] INTUBATED
- [ ] VENTILATOR
- [ ] TRACHEOSTOMY
- [ ] BIPAP / CPAP
- [ ] FACE MASK
- [ ] EXTUBATED
- [ ] HIGH FLOW
- [ ] NASAL PRONGS
- [ ] ROOM AIR
- [ ] OTHER

LEVEL OF CONSCIOUSNESS

- [ ] AWAKE
- [ ] ALERT
- [ ] ORIENTED
- [ ] PARALYTIC MEDICATION
- [ ] SEDATED
- [ ] LETHARGIC
- [ ] SEIZURE
- [ ] AGITATED
- [ ] HALLUCINATIONS
- [ ] CONFUSED
- [ ] DELIRIOUS
- [ ] OTHER

NUTRITION

- [ ] NOTHING BY MOUTH
- [ ] FEEDING TUBE
- [ ] FEEDS HELD
- [ ] TPN (IV)
- [ ] ICE CHIPS / CLEAR FLUIDS
- [ ] PUREED DIET
- [ ] REGULAR
- [ ] OTHER

WOUNDS / INJURIES

....

DAILY PROGRESS AND GOALS

EACH DAY, THERE MAY BE ONE OR MORE GOALS OF CARE THAT THE TEAM IS HOPING THE PATIENT WILL ACHIEVE.

....

NOTES

....

TESTS PERFORMED TODAY

☐ X-RAY ☐ BLOOD TESTS

☐ CT SCAN ☐ BREATHING TRIAL

☐ MRI ☐ SPUTUM / LUNG

☐ ULTRASOUND ☐ OTHER

TODAY'S EXERCISES

☐ RANGE OF MOTION ☐ SIT IN CHAIR

☐ REPOSITIONING ☐ BICYCLE

☐ SIT AT BEDSIDE ☐ WALKING

☐ STAND AT BEDSIDE ☐ BEDREST

INTERDISCIPLINARY ROUNDS

WHAT ARE THE MAJOR ISSUES / CONCERNS TODAY? IS THE PATIENT GETTING BETTER OR WORSE? WHAT ARE SHORT- & LONG-TERM GOALS?

....

....

....

TODAY YOU (PATIENT) FELT:

😠 ANGRY   🙁 TIRED   😕 SAD   🙂 HAPPY   😆 EXCITED   😴 SEDATED

BECAUSE: ☐ OTHER

1. ....

2. ....

3. ....

TODAY I (CAREGIVER) FELT:

😠 ANGRY   🙁 TIRED   😕 SAD   🙂 HAPPY   😆 EXCITED

BECAUSE: ☐ OTHER

1. ....

2. ....

3. ....

WHAT HAPPENED TODAY?

PATIENT EVENTS | NEWS | MAJOR WORLD EVENTS | FAMILY EVENTS | VISITORS | ACTIVITIES | ICU ENVIRONMENT | SOUNDS | LIFE UPDATES | HOLIDAYS | RECOVERY MILESTONE

....

....

....

....

....

TODAY WE ARE GRATEFUL FOR...

1. ....

2. ....

3. ....

TODAY'S MESSAGE OF HOPE

....

....

....

QUOTE OF THE DAY

"Some days there won't be a song in your heart. Sing anyways." - Emory Austin

TODAY'S ENTRY IS COMPLETED BY: ....

T H E R A P E U T I C
JOURNAL

TODAY'S DATE: ....

ROOM #: ....

ICU PHYSICIAN: ....

DAY NURSE: ....

NIGHT NURSE: ....

NUMBER OF IV PUMPS

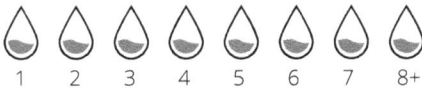

◇ ◇ ◇ ◇ ◇ ◇ ◇ ◇
1 2 3 4 5 6 7 8+

IV LINES

☐ IV LINE   ☐ INTRAOSSEOUS
☐ CENTRAL LINE   ☐ PORT
☐ PICC LINE   ☐ OTHER
☐ DIALYSIS LINE

BREATHING SUPPORT

☐ INTUBATED   ☐ EXTUBATED
☐ VENTILATOR   ☐ HIGH FLOW
☐ TRACHEOSTOMY   ☐ NASAL PRONGS
☐ BIPAP / CPAP   ☐ ROOM AIR
☐ FACE MASK   ☐ OTHER

LEVEL OF CONSCIOUSNESS

☐ AWAKE   ☐ SEIZURE
☐ ALERT   ☐ AGITATED
☐ ORIENTED   ☐ HALLUCINATIONS
☐ PARALYTIC MEDICATION   ☐ CONFUSED
☐ SEDATED   ☐ DELIRIOUS
☐ LETHARGIC   ☐ OTHER

NUTRITION

☐ NOTHING BY MOUTH   ☐ ICE CHIPS / CLEAR FLUIDS
☐ FEEDING TUBE   ☐ PUREED DIET
☐ FEEDS HELD   ☐ REGULAR
☐ TPN (IV)   ☐ OTHER

WOUNDS / INJURIES

....
....

DAILY PROGRESS AND GOALS

EACH DAY, THERE MAY BE ONE OR MORE GOALS OF CARE THAT THE TEAM IS HOPING THE PATIENT WILL ACHIEVE.

....
....

NOTES

....
....
....

TESTS PERFORMED TODAY

☐ X-RAY   ☐ BLOOD TESTS

☐ CT SCAN   ☐ BREATHING TRIAL

☐ MRI   ☐ SPUTUM / LUNG

☐ ULTRASOUND   ☐ OTHER

INTERDISCIPLINARY ROUNDS

TODAY'S EXERCISES

☐ RANGE OF MOTION   ☐ SIT IN CHAIR

☐ REPOSITIONING   ☐ BICYCLE

☐ SIT AT BEDSIDE   ☐ WALKING

☐ STAND AT BEDSIDE   ☐ BEDREST

WHAT ARE THE MAJOR ISSUES / CONCERNS TODAY? IS THE PATIENT GETTING BETTER OR WORSE? WHAT ARE SHORT- & LONG-TERM GOALS?

TODAY YOU (PATIENT) FELT:

ANGRY   TIRED   SAD   HAPPY   EXCITED   SEDATED

BECAUSE: ☐ OTHER

1.

2.

3.

TODAY I (CAREGIVER) FELT:

ANGRY   TIRED   SAD   HAPPY   EXCITED

BECAUSE: ☐ OTHER

1.

2.

3.

WHAT HAPPENED TODAY?

PATIENT EVENTS | NEWS | MAJOR WORLD EVENTS | FAMILY EVENTS | VISITORS | ACTIVITIES | ICU ENVIRONMENT | SOUNDS | LIFE UPDATES | HOLIDAYS | RECOVERY MILESTONE

TODAY WE ARE GRATEFUL FOR...

1.

2.

3.

TODAY'S MESSAGE OF HOPE

QUOTE OF THE DAY

"Strength does not come from physical capacity. It comes from indomitable will." - Mahatma Gandhi

TODAY'S ENTRY IS COMPLETED BY: ....

THERAPEUTIC
JOURNAL

TODAY'S DATE: ....

ROOM #: ....

ICU PHYSICIAN: ....

DAY NURSE: ....

NIGHT NURSE: ....

NUMBER OF IV PUMPS

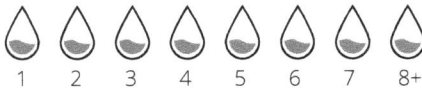

💧 💧 💧 💧 💧 💧 💧 💧
1 2 3 4 5 6 7 8+

IV LINES

- ☐ IV LINE
- ☐ CENTRAL LINE
- ☐ PICC LINE
- ☐ DIALYSIS LINE
- ☐ INTRAOSSEOUS
- ☐ PORT
- ☐ OTHER

BREATHING SUPPORT

- ☐ INTUBATED
- ☐ VENTILATOR
- ☐ TRACHEOSTOMY
- ☐ BIPAP / CPAP
- ☐ FACE MASK
- ☐ EXTUBATED
- ☐ HIGH FLOW
- ☐ NASAL PRONGS
- ☐ ROOM AIR
- ☐ OTHER

DAILY PROGRESS AND GOALS

LEVEL OF CONSCIOUSNESS

- ☐ AWAKE
- ☐ ALERT
- ☐ ORIENTED
- ☐ PARALYTIC MEDICATION
- ☐ SEDATED
- ☐ LETHARGIC
- ☐ SEIZURE
- ☐ AGITATED
- ☐ HALLUCINATIONS
- ☐ CONFUSED
- ☐ DELIRIOUS
- ☐ OTHER

NUTRITION

- ☐ NOTHING BY MOUTH
- ☐ FEEDING TUBE
- ☐ FEEDS HELD
- ☐ TPN (IV)
- ☐ ICE CHIPS / CLEAR FLUIDS
- ☐ PUREED DIET
- ☐ REGULAR
- ☐ OTHER

WOUNDS / INJURIES

....

....

EACH DAY, THERE MAY BE ONE OR MORE
GOALS OF CARE THAT THE TEAM IS HOPING THE
PATIENT WILL ACHIEVE.

....

....

NOTES

....

....

....

TESTS PERFORMED TODAY

- ☐ X-RAY
- ☐ CT SCAN
- ☐ MRI
- ☐ ULTRASOUND
- ☐ BLOOD TESTS
- ☐ BREATHING TRIAL
- ☐ SPUTUM / LUNG
- ☐ OTHER

TODAY'S EXERCISES

- ☐ RANGE OF MOTION
- ☐ REPOSITIONING
- ☐ SIT AT BEDSIDE
- ☐ STAND AT BEDSIDE
- ☐ SIT IN CHAIR
- ☐ BICYCLE
- ☐ WALKING
- ☐ BEDREST

INTERDISCIPLINARY ROUNDS

WHAT ARE THE MAJOR ISSUES / CONCERNS TODAY? IS THE PATIENT GETTING BETTER OR WORSE? WHAT ARE SHORT- & LONG-TERM GOALS?

TODAY YOU (PATIENT) FELT:

ANGRY   TIRED   SAD   HAPPY   EXCITED   SEDATED

BECAUSE: ☐ OTHER

1.
2.
3.

TODAY I (CAREGIVER) FELT:

ANGRY   TIRED   SAD   HAPPY   EXCITED

BECAUSE: ☐ OTHER

1.
2.
3.

WHAT HAPPENED TODAY?

PATIENT EVENTS | NEWS | MAJOR WORLD EVENTS | FAMILY EVENTS | VISITORS | ACTIVITIES | ICU ENVIRONMENT | SOUNDS | LIFE UPDATES | HOLIDAYS | RECOVERY MILESTONE

TODAY WE ARE GRATEFUL FOR...

1.
2.
3.

TODAY'S MESSAGE OF HOPE

QUOTE OF THE DAY

"The flower that blooms in adversity is the most rare and beautiful of all." - Fa Zhou

TODAY'S ENTRY IS COMPLETED BY: ....

T H E R A P E U T I C
J O U R N A L

TODAY'S DATE: ....

ROOM #: ....

ICU PHYSICIAN: ....

DAY NURSE: ....

NIGHT NURSE: ....

NUMBER OF IV PUMPS

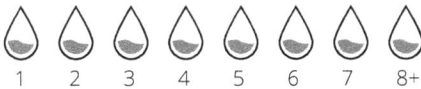

◇ ◇ ◇ ◇ ◇ ◇ ◇ ◇
1   2   3   4   5   6   7   8+

IV LINES

☐ IV LINE   ☐ INTRAOSSEOUS
☐ CENTRAL LINE   ☐ PORT
☐ PICC LINE   ☐ OTHER
☐ DIALYSIS LINE

BREATHING SUPPORT

☐ INTUBATED   ☐ EXTUBATED
☐ VENTILATOR   ☐ HIGH FLOW
☐ TRACHEOSTOMY   ☐ NASAL PRONGS
☐ BIPAP / CPAP   ☐ ROOM AIR
☐ FACE MASK   ☐ OTHER

LEVEL OF CONSCIOUSNESS

☐ AWAKE   ☐ SEIZURE
☐ ALERT   ☐ AGITATED
☐ ORIENTED   ☐ HALLUCINATIONS
☐ PARALYTIC MEDICATION   ☐ CONFUSED
☐ SEDATED   ☐ DELIRIOUS
☐ LETHARGIC   ☐ OTHER

NUTRITION

☐ NOTHING BY MOUTH   ☐ ICE CHIPS / CLEAR FLUIDS
☐ FEEDING TUBE   ☐ PUREED DIET
☐ FEEDS HELD   ☐ REGULAR
☐ TPN (IV)   ☐ OTHER

WOUNDS / INJURIES

....

....

DAILY PROGRESS AND GOALS

EACH DAY, THERE MAY BE ONE OR MORE
GOALS OF CARE THAT THE TEAM IS HOPING THE
PATIENT WILL ACHIEVE.

....

....

NOTES

....

....

....

TESTS PERFORMED TODAY

- ☐ X-RAY
- ☐ CT SCAN
- ☐ MRI
- ☐ ULTRASOUND
- ☐ BLOOD TESTS
- ☐ BREATHING TRIAL
- ☐ SPUTUM / LUNG
- ☐ OTHER

INTERDISCIPLINARY ROUNDS

TODAY'S EXERCISES

- ☐ RANGE OF MOTION
- ☐ REPOSITIONING
- ☐ SIT AT BEDSIDE
- ☐ STAND AT BEDSIDE
- ☐ SIT IN CHAIR
- ☐ BICYCLE
- ☐ WALKING
- ☐ BEDREST

WHAT ARE THE MAJOR ISSUES / CONCERNS TODAY? IS THE PATIENT GETTING BETTER OR WORSE? WHAT ARE SHORT- & LONG-TERM GOALS?

TODAY YOU (PATIENT) FELT:

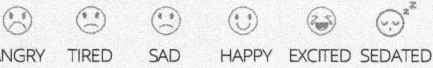

ANGRY   TIRED   SAD   HAPPY   EXCITED   SEDATED

BECAUSE: ☐ OTHER

1.
2.
3.

TODAY I (CAREGIVER) FELT:

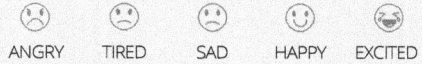

ANGRY   TIRED   SAD   HAPPY   EXCITED

BECAUSE: ☐ OTHER

1.
2.
3.

WHAT HAPPENED TODAY?

PATIENT EVENTS | NEWS | MAJOR WORLD EVENTS | FAMILY EVENTS | VISITORS | ACTIVITIES | ICU ENVIRONMENT | SOUNDS | LIFE UPDATES | HOLIDAYS | RECOVERY MILESTONE

TODAY WE ARE GRATEFUL FOR...

1.
2.
3.

TODAY'S MESSAGE OF HOPE

QUOTE OF THE DAY

"Eventually you will come to understand that love heals everything, and love is all there is." - Gary Zukav

TODAY'S ENTRY IS COMPLETED BY: ....

THERAPEUTIC
JOURNAL

TODAY'S DATE: ....

ROOM #: ....

ICU PHYSICIAN: ....

DAY NURSE: ....

NIGHT NURSE: ....

NUMBER OF IV PUMPS

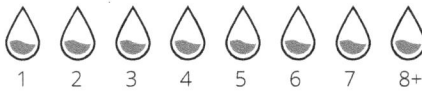

💧 💧 💧 💧 💧 💧 💧 💧
1   2   3   4   5   6   7   8+

IV LINES

☐ IV LINE   ☐ INTRAOSSEOUS
☐ CENTRAL LINE   ☐ PORT
☐ PICC LINE   ☐ OTHER
☐ DIALYSIS LINE

BREATHING SUPPORT

☐ INTUBATED   ☐ EXTUBATED
☐ VENTILATOR   ☐ HIGH FLOW
☐ TRACHEOSTOMY   ☐ NASAL PRONGS
☐ BIPAP / CPAP   ☐ ROOM AIR
☐ FACE MASK   ☐ OTHER

LEVEL OF CONSCIOUSNESS

☐ AWAKE   ☐ SEIZURE
☐ ALERT   ☐ AGITATED
☐ ORIENTED   ☐ HALLUCINATIONS
☐ PARALYTIC MEDICATION   ☐ CONFUSED
☐ SEDATED   ☐ DELIRIOUS
☐ LETHARGIC   ☐ OTHER

NUTRITION

☐ NOTHING BY MOUTH   ☐ ICE CHIPS / CLEAR FLUIDS
☐ FEEDING TUBE   ☐ PUREED DIET
☐ FEEDS HELD   ☐ REGULAR
☐ TPN (IV)   ☐ OTHER

WOUNDS / INJURIES

....
....

DAILY PROGRESS AND GOALS

EACH DAY, THERE MAY BE ONE OR MORE GOALS OF CARE THAT THE TEAM IS HOPING THE PATIENT WILL ACHIEVE.

....
....

NOTES

....
....
....

TESTS PERFORMED TODAY

☐ X-RAY   ☐ BLOOD TESTS

☐ CT SCAN   ☐ BREATHING TRIAL

☐ MRI   ☐ SPUTUM / LUNG

☐ ULTRASOUND   ☐ OTHER

INTERDISCIPLINARY ROUNDS

TODAY'S EXERCISES

☐ RANGE OF MOTION   ☐ SIT IN CHAIR

☐ REPOSITIONING   ☐ BICYCLE

☐ SIT AT BEDSIDE   ☐ WALKING

☐ STAND AT BEDSIDE   ☐ BEDREST

WHAT ARE THE MAJOR ISSUES / CONCERNS TODAY? IS THE PATIENT GETTING BETTER OR WORSE? WHAT ARE SHORT- & LONG-TERM GOALS?

TODAY YOU (PATIENT) FELT:

ANGRY   TIRED   SAD   HAPPY   EXCITED   SEDATED

BECAUSE: ☐ OTHER

1.

2.

3.

TODAY I (CAREGIVER) FELT:

ANGRY   TIRED   SAD   HAPPY   EXCITED

BECAUSE: ☐ OTHER

1.

2.

3.

WHAT HAPPENED TODAY?

PATIENT EVENTS | NEWS | MAJOR WORLD EVENTS | FAMILY EVENTS | VISITORS | ACTIVITIES | ICU ENVIRONMENT | SOUNDS | LIFE UPDATES | HOLIDAYS | RECOVERY MILESTONE

TODAY WE ARE GRATEFUL FOR...

1.

2.

3.

TODAY'S MESSAGE OF HOPE

QUOTE OF THE DAY

"The forces that are for you are greater than the forces against you." - Joel Osteen

TODAY'S ENTRY IS COMPLETED BY: ....

T H E R A P E U T I C
J O U R N A L

TODAY'S DATE: ....

ROOM #: ....

ICU PHYSICIAN: ....

DAY NURSE: ....

NIGHT NURSE: ....

NUMBER OF IV PUMPS

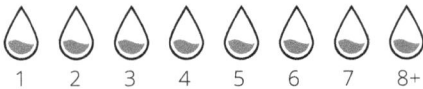

◇ ◇ ◇ ◇ ◇ ◇ ◇ ◇
1 2 3 4 5 6 7 8+

IV LINES

☐ IV LINE   ☐ INTRAOSSEOUS
☐ CENTRAL LINE   ☐ PORT
☐ PICC LINE   ☐ OTHER
☐ DIALYSIS LINE

BREATHING SUPPORT

☐ INTUBATED   ☐ EXTUBATED
☐ VENTILATOR   ☐ HIGH FLOW
☐ TRACHEOSTOMY   ☐ NASAL PRONGS
☐ BIPAP / CPAP   ☐ ROOM AIR
☐ FACE MASK   ☐ OTHER

LEVEL OF CONSCIOUSNESS

☐ AWAKE   ☐ SEIZURE
☐ ALERT   ☐ AGITATED
☐ ORIENTED   ☐ HALLUCINATIONS
☐ PARALYTIC MEDICATION   ☐ CONFUSED
☐ SEDATED   ☐ DELIRIOUS
☐ LETHARGIC   ☐ OTHER

NUTRITION

☐ NOTHING BY MOUTH   ☐ ICE CHIPS / CLEAR FLUIDS
☐ FEEDING TUBE   ☐ PUREED DIET
☐ FEEDS HELD   ☐ REGULAR
☐ TPN (IV)   ☐ OTHER

WOUNDS / INJURIES

....

....

DAILY PROGRESS AND GOALS

EACH DAY, THERE MAY BE ONE OR MORE GOALS OF CARE THAT THE TEAM IS HOPING THE PATIENT WILL ACHIEVE.

....

....

NOTES

....

....

....

TESTS PERFORMED TODAY

☐ X-RAY ☐ BLOOD TESTS

☐ CT SCAN ☐ BREATHING TRIAL

☐ MRI ☐ SPUTUM / LUNG

☐ ULTRASOUND ☐ OTHER

INTERDISCIPLINARY ROUNDS

TODAY'S EXERCISES

☐ RANGE OF MOTION ☐ SIT IN CHAIR

☐ REPOSITIONING ☐ BICYCLE

☐ SIT AT BEDSIDE ☐ WALKING

☐ STAND AT BEDSIDE ☐ BEDREST

WHAT ARE THE MAJOR ISSUES / CONCERNS TODAY? IS THE PATIENT GETTING BETTER OR WORSE? WHAT ARE SHORT- & LONG-TERM GOALS?

TODAY YOU (PATIENT) FELT:

ANGRY TIRED SAD HAPPY EXCITED SEDATED

BECAUSE: ☐ OTHER

1.

2.

3.

TODAY I (CAREGIVER) FELT:

ANGRY TIRED SAD HAPPY EXCITED

BECAUSE: ☐ OTHER

1.

2.

3.

WHAT HAPPENED TODAY?

PATIENT EVENTS | NEWS | MAJOR WORLD EVENTS | FAMILY EVENTS | VISITORS | ACTIVITIES | ICU ENVIRONMENT | SOUNDS | LIFE UPDATES | HOLIDAYS | RECOVERY MILESTONE

TODAY WE ARE GRATEFUL FOR...

1.

2.

3.

TODAY'S MESSAGE OF HOPE

QUOTE OF THE DAY

"Friends show their love in times of trouble, not in happiness." - Euripides

TODAY'S ENTRY IS COMPLETED BY: ....

T H E R A P E U T I C
J O U R N A L

TODAY'S DATE: ....

ROOM #: ....

ICU PHYSICIAN: ....

DAY NURSE: ....

NIGHT NURSE: ....

NUMBER OF IV PUMPS

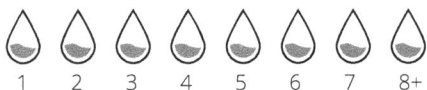

⬤ ⬤ ⬤ ⬤ ⬤ ⬤ ⬤ ⬤
1   2   3   4   5   6   7   8+

IV LINES

- ☐ IV LINE
- ☐ CENTRAL LINE
- ☐ PICC LINE
- ☐ DIALYSIS LINE
- ☐ INTRAOSSEOUS
- ☐ PORT
- ☐ OTHER

BREATHING SUPPORT

- ☐ INTUBATED
- ☐ VENTILATOR
- ☐ TRACHEOSTOMY
- ☐ BIPAP / CPAP
- ☐ FACE MASK
- ☐ EXTUBATED
- ☐ HIGH FLOW
- ☐ NASAL PRONGS
- ☐ ROOM AIR
- ☐ OTHER

LEVEL OF CONSCIOUSNESS

- ☐ AWAKE
- ☐ ALERT
- ☐ ORIENTED
- ☐ PARALYTIC MEDICATION
- ☐ SEDATED
- ☐ LETHARGIC
- ☐ SEIZURE
- ☐ AGITATED
- ☐ HALLUCINATIONS
- ☐ CONFUSED
- ☐ DELIRIOUS
- ☐ OTHER

NUTRITION

- ☐ NOTHING BY MOUTH
- ☐ FEEDING TUBE
- ☐ FEEDS HELD
- ☐ TPN (IV)
- ☐ ICE CHIPS / CLEAR FLUIDS
- ☐ PUREED DIET
- ☐ REGULAR
- ☐ OTHER

WOUNDS / INJURIES

....
....
....

DAILY PROGRESS AND GOALS

EACH DAY, THERE MAY BE ONE OR MORE GOALS OF CARE THAT THE TEAM IS HOPING THE PATIENT WILL ACHIEVE.

....
....

NOTES

....
....
....

TESTS PERFORMED TODAY

☐ X-RAY   ☐ BLOOD TESTS

☐ CT SCAN   ☐ BREATHING TRIAL

☐ MRI   ☐ SPUTUM / LUNG

☐ ULTRASOUND ☐ OTHER

INTERDISCIPLINARY ROUNDS

TODAY'S EXERCISES

☐ RANGE OF MOTION ☐ SIT IN CHAIR

☐ REPOSITIONING   ☐ BICYCLE

☐ SIT AT BEDSIDE   ☐ WALKING

☐ STAND AT BEDSIDE ☐ BEDREST

WHAT ARE THE MAJOR ISSUES / CONCERNS TODAY? IS THE PATIENT GETTING BETTER OR WORSE? WHAT ARE SHORT- & LONG-TERM GOALS?

....

....

....

....

TODAY YOU (PATIENT) FELT:

😠 ANGRY   🙁 TIRED   😐 SAD   🙂 HAPPY   😄 EXCITED   😴 SEDATED

BECAUSE: ☐ OTHER

1. ....

2. ....

3. ....

TODAY I (CAREGIVER) FELT:

😠 ANGRY   🙁 TIRED   😐 SAD   🙂 HAPPY   😄 EXCITED

BECAUSE: ☐ OTHER

1. ....

2. ....

3. ....

WHAT HAPPENED TODAY?

PATIENT EVENTS | NEWS | MAJOR WORLD EVENTS | FAMILY EVENTS | VISITORS | ACTIVITIES | ICU ENVIRONMENT | SOUNDS | LIFE UPDATES | HOLIDAYS | RECOVERY MILESTONE

....

....

....

....

....

....

TODAY WE ARE GRATEFUL FOR...

1. ....

2. ....

3. ....

TODAY'S MESSAGE OF HOPE

....

....

....

....

QUOTE OF THE DAY

"Being deeply loved by someone gives you strength, while loving someone deeply gives you courage." - Lao Tzu

TODAY'S ENTRY IS COMPLETED BY: ....

THERAPEUTIC
JOURNAL

TODAY'S DATE: ....

ROOM #: ....

ICU PHYSICIAN: ....

DAY NURSE: ....

NIGHT NURSE: ....

NUMBER OF IV PUMPS

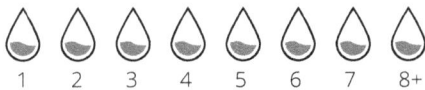

1   2   3   4   5   6   7   8+

IV LINES

☐ IV LINE
☐ CENTRAL LINE
☐ PICC LINE
☐ DIALYSIS LINE

☐ INTRAOSSEOUS
☐ PORT
☐ OTHER

BREATHING SUPPORT

☐ INTUBATED
☐ VENTILATOR
☐ TRACHEOSTOMY
☐ BIPAP / CPAP
☐ FACE MASK

☐ EXTUBATED
☐ HIGH FLOW
☐ NASAL PRONGS
☐ ROOM AIR
☐ OTHER

LEVEL OF CONSCIOUSNESS

☐ AWAKE
☐ ALERT
☐ ORIENTED
☐ PARALYTIC MEDICATION
☐ SEDATED
☐ LETHARGIC

☐ SEIZURE
☐ AGITATED
☐ HALLUCINATIONS
☐ CONFUSED
☐ DELIRIOUS
☐ OTHER

NUTRITION

☐ NOTHING BY MOUTH
☐ FEEDING TUBE
☐ FEEDS HELD
☐ TPN (IV)

☐ ICE CHIPS / CLEAR FLUIDS
☐ PUREED DIET
☐ REGULAR
☐ OTHER

WOUNDS / INJURIES

....

DAILY PROGRESS AND GOALS

EACH DAY, THERE MAY BE ONE OR MORE GOALS OF CARE THAT THE TEAM IS HOPING THE PATIENT WILL ACHIEVE.

....
....

NOTES

....
....
....

TESTS PERFORMED TODAY

☐ X-RAY   ☐ BLOOD TESTS

☐ CT SCAN   ☐ BREATHING TRIAL

☐ MRI   ☐ SPUTUM / LUNG

☐ ULTRASOUND   ☐ OTHER

TODAY'S EXERCISES

☐ RANGE OF MOTION   ☐ SIT IN CHAIR

☐ REPOSITIONING   ☐ BICYCLE

☐ SIT AT BEDSIDE   ☐ WALKING

☐ STAND AT BEDSIDE   ☐ BEDREST

INTERDISCIPLINARY ROUNDS

WHAT ARE THE MAJOR ISSUES / CONCERNS TODAY? IS THE PATIENT GETTING BETTER OR WORSE? WHAT ARE SHORT- & LONG-TERM GOALS?

TODAY YOU (PATIENT) FELT:

ANGRY   TIRED   SAD   HAPPY   EXCITED   SEDATED

BECAUSE: ☐ OTHER

1.

2.

3.

TODAY I (CAREGIVER) FELT:

ANGRY   TIRED   SAD   HAPPY   EXCITED

BECAUSE: ☐ OTHER

1.

2.

3.

WHAT HAPPENED TODAY?

PATIENT EVENTS | NEWS | MAJOR WORLD EVENTS | FAMILY EVENTS | VISITORS | ACTIVITIES | ICU ENVIRONMENT | SOUNDS | LIFE UPDATES | HOLIDAYS | RECOVERY MILESTONE

TODAY WE ARE GRATEFUL FOR...

1.

2.

3.

TODAY'S MESSAGE OF HOPE

QUOTE OF THE DAY

"Words of kindness are more healing to a dropping heart than balm or honey." - Sarah Fielding

TODAY'S ENTRY IS COMPLETED BY: ....

THERAPEUTIC
JOURNAL

ICU PHYSICIAN: ....

DAY NURSE: ....

NIGHT NURSE: ....

TODAY'S DATE: ....

ROOM #: ....

NUMBER OF IV PUMPS

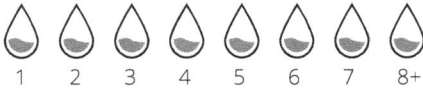

1 2 3 4 5 6 7 8+

IV LINES

- ☐ IV LINE
- ☐ CENTRAL LINE
- ☐ PICC LINE
- ☐ DIALYSIS LINE
- ☐ INTRAOSSEOUS
- ☐ PORT
- ☐ OTHER

BREATHING SUPPORT

- ☐ INTUBATED
- ☐ VENTILATOR
- ☐ TRACHEOSTOMY
- ☐ BIPAP / CPAP
- ☐ FACE MASK
- ☐ EXTUBATED
- ☐ HIGH FLOW
- ☐ NASAL PRONGS
- ☐ ROOM AIR
- ☐ OTHER

LEVEL OF CONSCIOUSNESS

- ☐ AWAKE
- ☐ ALERT
- ☐ ORIENTED
- ☐ PARALYTIC MEDICATION
- ☐ SEDATED
- ☐ LETHARGIC
- ☐ SEIZURE
- ☐ AGITATED
- ☐ HALLUCINATIONS
- ☐ CONFUSED
- ☐ DELIRIOUS
- ☐ OTHER

NUTRITION

- ☐ NOTHING BY MOUTH
- ☐ FEEDING TUBE
- ☐ FEEDS HELD
- ☐ TPN (IV)
- ☐ ICE CHIPS / CLEAR FLUIDS
- ☐ PUREED DIET
- ☐ REGULAR
- ☐ OTHER

WOUNDS / INJURIES

....

....

DAILY PROGRESS AND GOALS

EACH DAY, THERE MAY BE ONE OR MORE GOALS OF CARE THAT THE TEAM IS HOPING THE PATIENT WILL ACHIEVE.

....

....

NOTES

....

....

....

TESTS PERFORMED TODAY

- ☐ X-RAY
- ☐ CT SCAN
- ☐ MRI
- ☐ ULTRASOUND
- ☐ BLOOD TESTS
- ☐ BREATHING TRIAL
- ☐ SPUTUM / LUNG
- ☐ OTHER

TODAY'S EXERCISES

- ☐ RANGE OF MOTION
- ☐ REPOSITIONING
- ☐ SIT AT BEDSIDE
- ☐ STAND AT BEDSIDE
- ☐ SIT IN CHAIR
- ☐ BICYCLE
- ☐ WALKING
- ☐ BEDREST

INTERDISCIPLINARY ROUNDS

WHAT ARE THE MAJOR ISSUES / CONCERNS TODAY? IS THE PATIENT GETTING BETTER OR WORSE? WHAT ARE SHORT- & LONG-TERM GOALS?

....

....

....

....

TODAY YOU (PATIENT) FELT:

ANGRY   TIRED   SAD   HAPPY   EXCITED   SEDATED

BECAUSE: ☐ OTHER

1. ....

2. ....

3. ....

TODAY I (CAREGIVER) FELT:

ANGRY   TIRED   SAD   HAPPY   EXCITED

BECAUSE: ☐ OTHER

1. ....

2. ....

3. ....

WHAT HAPPENED TODAY?

PATIENT EVENTS | NEWS | MAJOR WORLD EVENTS | FAMILY EVENTS | VISITORS | ACTIVITIES | ICU ENVIRONMENT | SOUNDS | LIFE UPDATES | HOLIDAYS | RECOVERY MILESTONE

....

....

....

....

....

TODAY WE ARE GRATEFUL FOR...

1. ....

2. ....

3. ....

TODAY'S MESSAGE OF HOPE

....

....

....

....

QUOTE OF THE DAY

"The soul always knows what to do to heal itself. The challenge is to silence the mind." - Caroline Myss

TODAY'S ENTRY IS COMPLETED BY: _____

T H E R A P E U T I C
JOURNAL

TODAY'S DATE: _____

ROOM #: _____

ICU PHYSICIAN: _____

DAY NURSE: _____

NIGHT NURSE: _____

NUMBER OF IV PUMPS

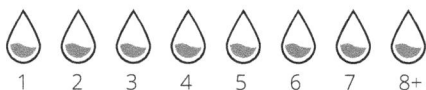

⬦ ⬦ ⬦ ⬦ ⬦ ⬦ ⬦ ⬦
1 2 3 4 5 6 7 8+

IV LINES

☐ IV LINE   ☐ INTRAOSSEOUS
☐ CENTRAL LINE   ☐ PORT
☐ PICC LINE   ☐ OTHER
☐ DIALYSIS LINE

BREATHING SUPPORT

☐ INTUBATED   ☐ EXTUBATED
☐ VENTILATOR   ☐ HIGH FLOW
☐ TRACHEOSTOMY   ☐ NASAL PRONGS
☐ BIPAP / CPAP   ☐ ROOM AIR
☐ FACE MASK   ☐ OTHER

LEVEL OF CONSCIOUSNESS

☐ AWAKE   ☐ SEIZURE
☐ ALERT   ☐ AGITATED
☐ ORIENTED   ☐ HALLUCINATIONS
☐ PARALYTIC MEDICATION   ☐ CONFUSED
☐ SEDATED   ☐ DELIRIOUS
☐ LETHARGIC   ☐ OTHER

NUTRITION

☐ NOTHING BY MOUTH   ☐ ICE CHIPS / CLEAR FLUIDS
☐ FEEDING TUBE   ☐ PUREED DIET
☐ FEEDS HELD   ☐ REGULAR
☐ TPN (IV)   ☐ OTHER

WOUNDS / INJURIES

_____

DAILY PROGRESS AND GOALS

EACH DAY, THERE MAY BE ONE OR MORE GOALS OF CARE THAT THE TEAM IS HOPING THE PATIENT WILL ACHIEVE.

_____

NOTES

_____

TESTS PERFORMED TODAY

- [ ] X-RAY
- [ ] BLOOD TESTS
- [ ] CT SCAN
- [ ] BREATHING TRIAL
- [ ] MRI
- [ ] SPUTUM / LUNG
- [ ] ULTRASOUND
- [ ] OTHER

INTERDISCIPLINARY ROUNDS

TODAY'S EXERCISES

- [ ] RANGE OF MOTION
- [ ] SIT IN CHAIR
- [ ] REPOSITIONING
- [ ] BICYCLE
- [ ] SIT AT BEDSIDE
- [ ] WALKING
- [ ] STAND AT BEDSIDE
- [ ] BEDREST

WHAT ARE THE MAJOR ISSUES / CONCERNS TODAY? IS THE PATIENT GETTING BETTER OR WORSE? WHAT ARE SHORT- & LONG-TERM GOALS?

TODAY YOU (PATIENT) FELT:

ANGRY   TIRED   SAD   HAPPY   EXCITED   SEDATED

BECAUSE: [ ] OTHER

1.
2.
3.

TODAY I (CAREGIVER) FELT:

ANGRY   TIRED   SAD   HAPPY   EXCITED

BECAUSE: [ ] OTHER

1.
2.
3.

WHAT HAPPENED TODAY?

PATIENT EVENTS | NEWS | MAJOR WORLD EVENTS | FAMILY EVENTS | VISITORS | ACTIVITIES | ICU ENVIRONMENT | SOUNDS | LIFE UPDATES | HOLIDAYS | RECOVERY MILESTONE

TODAY WE ARE GRATEFUL FOR...

1.
2.
3.

TODAY'S MESSAGE OF HOPE

QUOTE OF THE DAY

"Out of suffering have emerged the strongest souls; the most massive characters are seared with scars." - Khalil Gibran

TODAY'S ENTRY IS COMPLETED BY: ....

THERAPEUTIC
JOURNAL

TODAY'S DATE: ....

ROOM #: ....

ICU PHYSICIAN: ....

DAY NURSE: ....

NIGHT NURSE: ....

NUMBER OF IV PUMPS

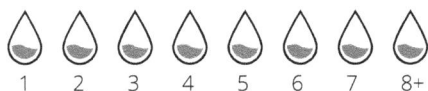

💧 💧 💧 💧 💧 💧 💧 💧
1   2   3   4   5   6   7   8+

IV LINES

- ☐ IV LINE
- ☐ CENTRAL LINE
- ☐ PICC LINE
- ☐ DIALYSIS LINE
- ☐ INTRAOSSEOUS
- ☐ PORT
- ☐ OTHER

BREATHING SUPPORT

- ☐ INTUBATED
- ☐ VENTILATOR
- ☐ TRACHEOSTOMY
- ☐ BIPAP / CPAP
- ☐ FACE MASK
- ☐ EXTUBATED
- ☐ HIGH FLOW
- ☐ NASAL PRONGS
- ☐ ROOM AIR
- ☐ OTHER

LEVEL OF CONSCIOUSNESS

- ☐ AWAKE
- ☐ ALERT
- ☐ ORIENTED
- ☐ PARALYTIC MEDICATION
- ☐ SEDATED
- ☐ LETHARGIC
- ☐ SEIZURE
- ☐ AGITATED
- ☐ HALLUCINATIONS
- ☐ CONFUSED
- ☐ DELIRIOUS
- ☐ OTHER

NUTRITION

- ☐ NOTHING BY MOUTH
- ☐ FEEDING TUBE
- ☐ FEEDS HELD
- ☐ TPN (IV)
- ☐ ICE CHIPS / CLEAR FLUIDS
- ☐ PUREED DIET
- ☐ REGULAR
- ☐ OTHER

WOUNDS / INJURIES

....
....

DAILY PROGRESS AND GOALS

EACH DAY, THERE MAY BE ONE OR MORE GOALS OF CARE THAT THE TEAM IS HOPING THE PATIENT WILL ACHIEVE.

....
....

NOTES

....
....
....

TESTS PERFORMED TODAY

☐ X-RAY   ☐ BLOOD TESTS

☐ CT SCAN   ☐ BREATHING TRIAL

☐ MRI   ☐ SPUTUM / LUNG

☐ ULTRASOUND   ☐ OTHER

INTERDISCIPLINARY ROUNDS

TODAY'S EXERCISES

☐ RANGE OF MOTION   ☐ SIT IN CHAIR

☐ REPOSITIONING   ☐ BICYCLE

☐ SIT AT BEDSIDE   ☐ WALKING

☐ STAND AT BEDSIDE   ☐ BEDREST

WHAT ARE THE MAJOR ISSUES / CONCERNS TODAY? IS
THE PATIENT GETTING BETTER OR WORSE? WHAT ARE
SHORT- & LONG-TERM GOALS?

TODAY YOU (PATIENT) FELT:

ANGRY   TIRED   SAD   HAPPY   EXCITED   SEDATED

BECAUSE: ☐ OTHER

1.

2.

3.

TODAY I (CAREGIVER) FELT:

ANGRY   TIRED   SAD   HAPPY   EXCITED

BECAUSE: ☐ OTHER

1.

2.

3.

WHAT HAPPENED TODAY?

PATIENT EVENTS | NEWS | MAJOR WORLD EVENTS | FAMILY
EVENTS | VISITORS | ACTIVITIES | ICU ENVIRONMENT |
SOUNDS | LIFE UPDATES | HOLIDAYS | RECOVERY MILESTONE

TODAY WE ARE GRATEFUL FOR...

1.

2.

3.

TODAY'S MESSAGE OF HOPE

QUOTE OF THE DAY

"I can be changed by what happens to me. But I refuse to be
reduced by it." - Maya Angelou

TODAY'S ENTRY IS COMPLETED BY: ....

THERAPEUTIC
JOURNAL

TODAY'S DATE: ....

ROOM #: ....

ICU PHYSICIAN: ....

DAY NURSE: ....

NIGHT NURSE: ....

NUMBER OF IV PUMPS

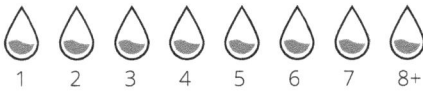

1 2 3 4 5 6 7 8+

IV LINES

- [ ] IV LINE
- [ ] CENTRAL LINE
- [ ] PICC LINE
- [ ] DIALYSIS LINE
- [ ] INTRAOSSEOUS
- [ ] PORT
- [ ] OTHER

BREATHING SUPPORT

- [ ] INTUBATED
- [ ] VENTILATOR
- [ ] TRACHEOSTOMY
- [ ] BIPAP / CPAP
- [ ] FACE MASK
- [ ] EXTUBATED
- [ ] HIGH FLOW
- [ ] NASAL PRONGS
- [ ] ROOM AIR
- [ ] OTHER

LEVEL OF CONSCIOUSNESS

- [ ] AWAKE
- [ ] ALERT
- [ ] ORIENTED
- [ ] PARALYTIC MEDICATION
- [ ] SEDATED
- [ ] LETHARGIC
- [ ] SEIZURE
- [ ] AGITATED
- [ ] HALLUCINATIONS
- [ ] CONFUSED
- [ ] DELIRIOUS
- [ ] OTHER

NUTRITION

- [ ] NOTHING BY MOUTH
- [ ] FEEDING TUBE
- [ ] FEEDS HELD
- [ ] TPN (IV)
- [ ] ICE CHIPS / CLEAR FLUIDS
- [ ] PUREED DIET
- [ ] REGULAR
- [ ] OTHER

WOUNDS / INJURIES

....

....

DAILY PROGRESS AND GOALS

EACH DAY, THERE MAY BE ONE OR MORE GOALS OF CARE THAT THE TEAM IS HOPING THE PATIENT WILL ACHIEVE.

....

....

NOTES

....

....

....

TESTS PERFORMED TODAY

- [ ] X-RAY
- [ ] CT SCAN
- [ ] MRI
- [ ] ULTRASOUND
- [ ] BLOOD TESTS
- [ ] BREATHING TRIAL
- [ ] SPUTUM / LUNG
- [ ] OTHER

INTERDISCIPLINARY ROUNDS

TODAY'S EXERCISES

- [ ] RANGE OF MOTION
- [ ] REPOSITIONING
- [ ] SIT AT BEDSIDE
- [ ] STAND AT BEDSIDE
- [ ] SIT IN CHAIR
- [ ] BICYCLE
- [ ] WALKING
- [ ] BEDREST

WHAT ARE THE MAJOR ISSUES / CONCERNS TODAY? IS THE PATIENT GETTING BETTER OR WORSE? WHAT ARE SHORT- & LONG-TERM GOALS?

TODAY YOU (PATIENT) FELT:

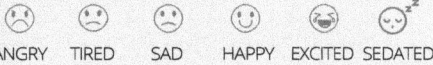

ANGRY   TIRED   SAD   HAPPY   EXCITED   SEDATED

BECAUSE: [ ] OTHER

1.
2.
3.

TODAY I (CAREGIVER) FELT:

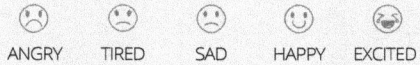

ANGRY   TIRED   SAD   HAPPY   EXCITED

BECAUSE: [ ] OTHER

1.
2.
3.

WHAT HAPPENED TODAY?

PATIENT EVENTS | NEWS | MAJOR WORLD EVENTS | FAMILY EVENTS | VISITORS | ACTIVITIES | ICU ENVIRONMENT | SOUNDS | LIFE UPDATES | HOLIDAYS | RECOVERY MILESTONE

TODAY WE ARE GRATEFUL FOR...

1.
2.
3.

TODAY'S MESSAGE OF HOPE

QUOTE OF THE DAY

"I sustain myself with the love of family." - Maya Angelou

TODAY'S ENTRY IS COMPLETED BY: ....

THERAPEUTIC
JOURNAL

TODAY'S DATE: ....

ROOM #: ....

ICU PHYSICIAN: ....

DAY NURSE: ....

NIGHT NURSE: ....

NUMBER OF IV PUMPS

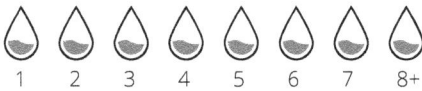

◊ ◊ ◊ ◊ ◊ ◊ ◊ ◊
1 2 3 4 5 6 7 8+

IV LINES

- [ ] IV LINE
- [ ] CENTRAL LINE
- [ ] PICC LINE
- [ ] DIALYSIS LINE
- [ ] INTRAOSSEOUS
- [ ] PORT
- [ ] OTHER

BREATHING SUPPORT

- [ ] INTUBATED
- [ ] VENTILATOR
- [ ] TRACHEOSTOMY
- [ ] BIPAP / CPAP
- [ ] FACE MASK
- [ ] EXTUBATED
- [ ] HIGH FLOW
- [ ] NASAL PRONGS
- [ ] ROOM AIR
- [ ] OTHER

LEVEL OF CONSCIOUSNESS

- [ ] AWAKE
- [ ] ALERT
- [ ] ORIENTED
- [ ] PARALYTIC MEDICATION
- [ ] SEDATED
- [ ] LETHARGIC
- [ ] SEIZURE
- [ ] AGITATED
- [ ] HALLUCINATIONS
- [ ] CONFUSED
- [ ] DELIRIOUS
- [ ] OTHER

NUTRITION

- [ ] NOTHING BY MOUTH
- [ ] FEEDING TUBE
- [ ] FEEDS HELD
- [ ] TPN (IV)
- [ ] ICE CHIPS / CLEAR FLUIDS
- [ ] PUREED DIET
- [ ] REGULAR
- [ ] OTHER

WOUNDS / INJURIES

DAILY PROGRESS AND GOALS

EACH DAY, THERE MAY BE ONE OR MORE GOALS OF CARE THAT THE TEAM IS HOPING THE PATIENT WILL ACHIEVE.

NOTES

TESTS PERFORMED TODAY

- ☐ X-RAY
- ☐ CT SCAN
- ☐ MRI
- ☐ ULTRASOUND
- ☐ BLOOD TESTS
- ☐ BREATHING TRIAL
- ☐ SPUTUM / LUNG
- ☐ OTHER

INTERDISCIPLINARY ROUNDS

TODAY'S EXERCISES

- ☐ RANGE OF MOTION
- ☐ REPOSITIONING
- ☐ SIT AT BEDSIDE
- ☐ STAND AT BEDSIDE
- ☐ SIT IN CHAIR
- ☐ BICYCLE
- ☐ WALKING
- ☐ BEDREST

WHAT ARE THE MAJOR ISSUES / CONCERNS TODAY? IS THE PATIENT GETTING BETTER OR WORSE? WHAT ARE SHORT- & LONG-TERM GOALS?

TODAY YOU (PATIENT) FELT:

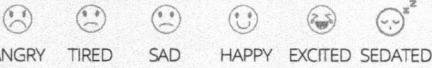

ANGRY   TIRED   SAD   HAPPY   EXCITED   SEDATED

BECAUSE: ☐ OTHER

1.
2.
3.

TODAY I (CAREGIVER) FELT:

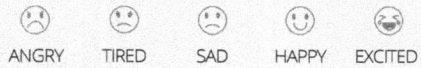

ANGRY   TIRED   SAD   HAPPY   EXCITED

BECAUSE: ☐ OTHER

1.
2.
3.

WHAT HAPPENED TODAY?

PATIENT EVENTS | NEWS | MAJOR WORLD EVENTS | FAMILY EVENTS | VISITORS | ACTIVITIES | ICU ENVIRONMENT | SOUNDS | LIFE UPDATES | HOLIDAYS | RECOVERY MILESTONE

TODAY WE ARE GRATEFUL FOR...

1.
2.
3.

TODAY'S MESSAGE OF HOPE

QUOTE OF THE DAY

"Once you choose hope, anything's possible."
- Christopher Reeve

TODAY'S ENTRY IS COMPLETED BY: ....

THERAPEUTIC
JOURNAL

TODAY'S DATE: ....

ROOM #: ....

ICU PHYSICIAN: ....

DAY NURSE: ....

NIGHT NURSE: ....

NUMBER OF IV PUMPS

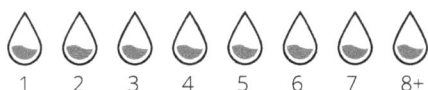

1 2 3 4 5 6 7 8+

IV LINES

- ☐ IV LINE
- ☐ CENTRAL LINE
- ☐ PICC LINE
- ☐ DIALYSIS LINE
- ☐ INTRAOSSEOUS
- ☐ PORT
- ☐ OTHER

BREATHING SUPPORT

- ☐ INTUBATED
- ☐ VENTILATOR
- ☐ TRACHEOSTOMY
- ☐ BIPAP / CPAP
- ☐ FACE MASK
- ☐ EXTUBATED
- ☐ HIGH FLOW
- ☐ NASAL PRONGS
- ☐ ROOM AIR
- ☐ OTHER

LEVEL OF CONSCIOUSNESS

- ☐ AWAKE
- ☐ ALERT
- ☐ ORIENTED
- ☐ PARALYTIC MEDICATION
- ☐ SEDATED
- ☐ LETHARGIC
- ☐ SEIZURE
- ☐ AGITATED
- ☐ HALLUCINATIONS
- ☐ CONFUSED
- ☐ DELIRIOUS
- ☐ OTHER

NUTRITION

- ☐ NOTHING BY MOUTH
- ☐ FEEDING TUBE
- ☐ FEEDS HELD
- ☐ TPN (IV)
- ☐ ICE CHIPS / CLEAR FLUIDS
- ☐ PUREED DIET
- ☐ REGULAR
- ☐ OTHER

WOUNDS / INJURIES

....

....

DAILY PROGRESS AND GOALS

EACH DAY, THERE MAY BE ONE OR MORE GOALS OF CARE THAT THE TEAM IS HOPING THE PATIENT WILL ACHIEVE.

....

....

NOTES

....

....

....

TESTS PERFORMED TODAY

☐ X-RAY   ☐ BLOOD TESTS

☐ CT SCAN   ☐ BREATHING TRIAL

☐ MRI   ☐ SPUTUM / LUNG

☐ ULTRASOUND   ☐ OTHER

INTERDISCIPLINARY ROUNDS

TODAY'S EXERCISES

☐ RANGE OF MOTION   ☐ SIT IN CHAIR

☐ REPOSITIONING   ☐ BICYCLE

☐ SIT AT BEDSIDE   ☐ WALKING

☐ STAND AT BEDSIDE ☐ BEDREST

WHAT ARE THE MAJOR ISSUES / CONCERNS TODAY? IS THE PATIENT GETTING BETTER OR WORSE? WHAT ARE SHORT- & LONG-TERM GOALS?

....

....

....

....

TODAY YOU (PATIENT) FELT:

ANGRY   TIRED   SAD   HAPPY   EXCITED   SEDATED

BECAUSE: ☐ OTHER

1. ....

2. ....

3. ....

TODAY I (CAREGIVER) FELT:

ANGRY   TIRED   SAD   HAPPY   EXCITED

BECAUSE: ☐ OTHER

1. ....

2. ....

3. ....

WHAT HAPPENED TODAY?

PATIENT EVENTS | NEWS | MAJOR WORLD EVENTS | FAMILY EVENTS | VISITORS | ACTIVITIES | ICU ENVIRONMENT | SOUNDS | LIFE UPDATES | HOLIDAYS | RECOVERY MILESTONE

....

....

....

....

....

....

....

TODAY WE ARE GRATEFUL FOR...

1. ....

2. ....

3. ....

TODAY'S MESSAGE OF HOPE

....

....

....

....

QUOTE OF THE DAY

"It's not the strength of the body that counts, but the strength of the spirit." - J.R.R. Tolkien

TODAY'S ENTRY IS COMPLETED BY: ....

THERAPEUTIC
JOURNAL

TODAY'S DATE: ....

ROOM #: ....

ICU PHYSICIAN: ....

DAY NURSE: ....

NIGHT NURSE: ....

NUMBER OF IV PUMPS

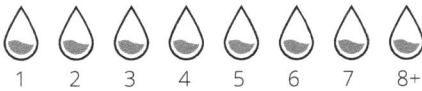

1 2 3 4 5 6 7 8+

IV LINES

- ☐ IV LINE
- ☐ CENTRAL LINE
- ☐ PICC LINE
- ☐ DIALYSIS LINE
- ☐ INTRAOSSEOUS
- ☐ PORT
- ☐ OTHER

BREATHING SUPPORT

- ☐ INTUBATED
- ☐ VENTILATOR
- ☐ TRACHEOSTOMY
- ☐ BIPAP / CPAP
- ☐ FACE MASK
- ☐ EXTUBATED
- ☐ HIGH FLOW
- ☐ NASAL PRONGS
- ☐ ROOM AIR
- ☐ OTHER

LEVEL OF CONSCIOUSNESS

- ☐ AWAKE
- ☐ ALERT
- ☐ ORIENTED
- ☐ PARALYTIC MEDICATION
- ☐ SEDATED
- ☐ LETHARGIC
- ☐ SEIZURE
- ☐ AGITATED
- ☐ HALLUCINATIONS
- ☐ CONFUSED
- ☐ DELIRIOUS
- ☐ OTHER

NUTRITION

- ☐ NOTHING BY MOUTH
- ☐ FEEDING TUBE
- ☐ FEEDS HELD
- ☐ TPN (IV)
- ☐ ICE CHIPS / CLEAR FLUIDS
- ☐ PUREED DIET
- ☐ REGULAR
- ☐ OTHER

WOUNDS / INJURIES

....

....

DAILY PROGRESS AND GOALS

EACH DAY, THERE MAY BE ONE OR MORE GOALS OF CARE THAT THE TEAM IS HOPING THE PATIENT WILL ACHIEVE.

....

....

NOTES

....

....

....

TESTS PERFORMED TODAY

- ☐ X-RAY
- ☐ CT SCAN
- ☐ MRI
- ☐ ULTRASOUND
- ☐ BLOOD TESTS
- ☐ BREATHING TRIAL
- ☐ SPUTUM / LUNG
- ☐ OTHER

INTERDISCIPLINARY ROUNDS

TODAY'S EXERCISES

- ☐ RANGE OF MOTION
- ☐ REPOSITIONING
- ☐ SIT AT BEDSIDE
- ☐ STAND AT BEDSIDE
- ☐ SIT IN CHAIR
- ☐ BICYCLE
- ☐ WALKING
- ☐ BEDREST

WHAT ARE THE MAJOR ISSUES / CONCERNS TODAY? IS THE PATIENT GETTING BETTER OR WORSE? WHAT ARE SHORT- & LONG-TERM GOALS?

TODAY YOU (PATIENT) FELT:

ANGRY   TIRED   SAD   HAPPY   EXCITED   SEDATED

BECAUSE: ☐ OTHER

1.
2.
3.

TODAY I (CAREGIVER) FELT:

ANGRY   TIRED   SAD   HAPPY   EXCITED

BECAUSE: ☐ OTHER

1.
2.
3.

WHAT HAPPENED TODAY?

PATIENT EVENTS | NEWS | MAJOR WORLD EVENTS | FAMILY EVENTS | VISITORS | ACTIVITIES | ICU ENVIRONMENT | SOUNDS | LIFE UPDATES | HOLIDAYS | RECOVERY MILESTONE

TODAY WE ARE GRATEFUL FOR...

1.
2.
3.

TODAY'S MESSAGE OF HOPE

QUOTE OF THE DAY

"Character cannot be developed in ease and quiet. Only through experience of trial and suffering can the soul be strengthened, ambition inspired, and success achieved."
- Helen Keller

TODAY'S ENTRY IS COMPLETED BY: ....

THERAPEUTIC
JOURNAL

TODAY'S DATE: ....

ROOM #: ....

ICU PHYSICIAN: ....

DAY NURSE: ....

NIGHT NURSE: ....

NUMBER OF IV PUMPS

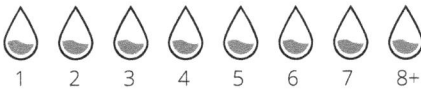

◊ ◊ ◊ ◊ ◊ ◊ ◊ ◊
1 2 3 4 5 6 7 8+

IV LINES

☐ IV LINE   ☐ INTRAOSSEOUS
☐ CENTRAL LINE   ☐ PORT
☐ PICC LINE   ☐ OTHER
☐ DIALYSIS LINE

BREATHING SUPPORT

☐ INTUBATED   ☐ EXTUBATED
☐ VENTILATOR   ☐ HIGH FLOW
☐ TRACHEOSTOMY   ☐ NASAL PRONGS
☐ BIPAP / CPAP   ☐ ROOM AIR
☐ FACE MASK   ☐ OTHER

DAILY PROGRESS AND GOALS

LEVEL OF CONSCIOUSNESS

☐ AWAKE   ☐ SEIZURE
☐ ALERT   ☐ AGITATED
☐ ORIENTED   ☐ HALLUCINATIONS
☐ PARALYTIC MEDICATION   ☐ CONFUSED
☐ SEDATED   ☐ DELIRIOUS
☐ LETHARGIC   ☐ OTHER

NUTRITION

☐ NOTHING BY MOUTH   ☐ ICE CHIPS / CLEAR FLUIDS
☐ FEEDING TUBE   ☐ PUREED DIET
☐ FEEDS HELD   ☐ REGULAR
☐ TPN (IV)   ☐ OTHER

WOUNDS / INJURIES

....

....

EACH DAY, THERE MAY BE ONE OR MORE
GOALS OF CARE THAT THE TEAM IS HOPING THE
PATIENT WILL ACHIEVE.

NOTES

....

....

....

TESTS PERFORMED TODAY

☐ X-RAY   ☐ BLOOD TESTS

☐ CT SCAN   ☐ BREATHING TRIAL

☐ MRI   ☐ SPUTUM / LUNG

☐ ULTRASOUND   ☐ OTHER

INTERDISCIPLINARY ROUNDS

TODAY'S EXERCISES

☐ RANGE OF MOTION   ☐ SIT IN CHAIR

☐ REPOSITIONING   ☐ BICYCLE

☐ SIT AT BEDSIDE   ☐ WALKING

☐ STAND AT BEDSIDE   ☐ BEDREST

WHAT ARE THE MAJOR ISSUES / CONCERNS TODAY? IS THE PATIENT GETTING BETTER OR WORSE? WHAT ARE SHORT- & LONG-TERM GOALS?

TODAY YOU (PATIENT) FELT:

😠   😔   😟   😊   😄   😴

ANGRY   TIRED   SAD   HAPPY   EXCITED   SEDATED

BECAUSE: ☐ OTHER

1.

2.

3.

TODAY I (CAREGIVER) FELT:

😠   😔   😟   😊   😄

ANGRY   TIRED   SAD   HAPPY   EXCITED

BECAUSE: ☐ OTHER

1.

2.

3.

WHAT HAPPENED TODAY?

PATIENT EVENTS | NEWS | MAJOR WORLD EVENTS | FAMILY EVENTS | VISITORS | ACTIVITIES | ICU ENVIRONMENT | SOUNDS | LIFE UPDATES | HOLIDAYS | RECOVERY MILESTONE

TODAY WE ARE GRATEFUL FOR...

1.

2.

3.

TODAY'S MESSAGE OF HOPE

QUOTE OF THE DAY

"Every day may not be good, but there's something good in every day. Focus on the good, no matter how small."
- Alice Morse Earle

TODAY'S ENTRY IS COMPLETED BY: ....

THERAPEUTIC
JOURNAL

TODAY'S DATE: ....

ROOM #: ....

ICU PHYSICIAN: ....

DAY NURSE: ....

NIGHT NURSE: ....

NUMBER OF IV PUMPS

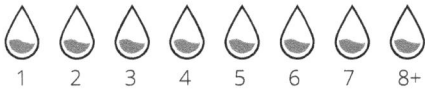

1   2   3   4   5   6   7   8+

IV LINES

- ☐ IV LINE
- ☐ CENTRAL LINE
- ☐ PICC LINE
- ☐ DIALYSIS LINE
- ☐ INTRAOSSEOUS
- ☐ PORT
- ☐ OTHER

BREATHING SUPPORT

- ☐ INTUBATED
- ☐ VENTILATOR
- ☐ TRACHEOSTOMY
- ☐ BIPAP / CPAP
- ☐ FACE MASK
- ☐ EXTUBATED
- ☐ HIGH FLOW
- ☐ NASAL PRONGS
- ☐ ROOM AIR
- ☐ OTHER

LEVEL OF CONSCIOUSNESS

- ☐ AWAKE
- ☐ ALERT
- ☐ ORIENTED
- ☐ PARALYTIC MEDICATION
- ☐ SEDATED
- ☐ LETHARGIC
- ☐ SEIZURE
- ☐ AGITATED
- ☐ HALLUCINATIONS
- ☐ CONFUSED
- ☐ DELIRIOUS
- ☐ OTHER

NUTRITION

- ☐ NOTHING BY MOUTH
- ☐ FEEDING TUBE
- ☐ FEEDS HELD
- ☐ TPN (IV)
- ☐ ICE CHIPS / CLEAR FLUIDS
- ☐ PUREED DIET
- ☐ REGULAR
- ☐ OTHER

WOUNDS / INJURIES

....

....

DAILY PROGRESS AND GOALS

EACH DAY, THERE MAY BE ONE OR MORE GOALS OF CARE THAT THE TEAM IS HOPING THE PATIENT WILL ACHIEVE.

....

....

NOTES

....

....

....

TESTS PERFORMED TODAY

- ☐ X-RAY
- ☐ CT SCAN
- ☐ MRI
- ☐ ULTRASOUND
- ☐ BLOOD TESTS
- ☐ BREATHING TRIAL
- ☐ SPUTUM / LUNG
- ☐ OTHER

INTERDISCIPLINARY ROUNDS

TODAY'S EXERCISES

- ☐ RANGE OF MOTION
- ☐ REPOSITIONING
- ☐ SIT AT BEDSIDE
- ☐ STAND AT BEDSIDE
- ☐ SIT IN CHAIR
- ☐ BICYCLE
- ☐ WALKING
- ☐ BEDREST

WHAT ARE THE MAJOR ISSUES / CONCERNS TODAY? IS THE PATIENT GETTING BETTER OR WORSE? WHAT ARE SHORT- & LONG-TERM GOALS?

TODAY YOU (PATIENT) FELT:

ANGRY   TIRED   SAD   HAPPY   EXCITED   SEDATED

BECAUSE: ☐ OTHER

1.
2.
3.

TODAY I (CAREGIVER) FELT:

ANGRY   TIRED   SAD   HAPPY   EXCITED

BECAUSE: ☐ OTHER

1.
2.
3.

WHAT HAPPENED TODAY?

PATIENT EVENTS | NEWS | MAJOR WORLD EVENTS | FAMILY EVENTS | VISITORS | ACTIVITIES | ICU ENVIRONMENT | SOUNDS | LIFE UPDATES | HOLIDAYS | RECOVERY MILESTONE

TODAY WE ARE GRATEFUL FOR...

1.
2.
3.

TODAY'S MESSAGE OF HOPE

QUOTE OF THE DAY

"No matter how much falls on us, we keep ploughing ahead. That's the only way to keep the roads clear." - Greg Kincaid

TODAY'S ENTRY IS COMPLETED BY: ....

THERAPEUTIC
JOURNAL

TODAY'S DATE: ....

ROOM #: ....

ICU PHYSICIAN: ....

DAY NURSE: ....

NIGHT NURSE: ....

NUMBER OF IV PUMPS

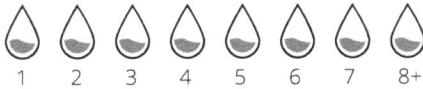

1   2   3   4   5   6   7   8+

IV LINES

☐ IV LINE   ☐ INTRAOSSEOUS
☐ CENTRAL LINE   ☐ PORT
☐ PICC LINE   ☐ OTHER
☐ DIALYSIS LINE

BREATHING SUPPORT

☐ INTUBATED   ☐ EXTUBATED
☐ VENTILATOR   ☐ HIGH FLOW
☐ TRACHEOSTOMY   ☐ NASAL PRONGS
☐ BIPAP / CPAP   ☐ ROOM AIR
☐ FACE MASK   ☐ OTHER

LEVEL OF CONSCIOUSNESS

☐ AWAKE   ☐ SEIZURE
☐ ALERT   ☐ AGITATED
☐ ORIENTED   ☐ HALLUCINATIONS
☐ PARALYTIC MEDICATION   ☐ CONFUSED
☐ SEDATED   ☐ DELIRIOUS
☐ LETHARGIC   ☐ OTHER

NUTRITION

☐ NOTHING BY MOUTH   ☐ ICE CHIPS / CLEAR FLUIDS
☐ FEEDING TUBE   ☐ PUREED DIET
☐ FEEDS HELD   ☐ REGULAR
☐ TPN (IV)   ☐ OTHER

WOUNDS / INJURIES

....

DAILY PROGRESS AND GOALS

EACH DAY, THERE MAY BE ONE OR MORE GOALS OF CARE THAT THE TEAM IS HOPING THE PATIENT WILL ACHIEVE.

....
....

NOTES

....
....
....

TESTS PERFORMED TODAY

☐ X-RAY   ☐ BLOOD TESTS

☐ CT SCAN   ☐ BREATHING TRIAL

☐ MRI   ☐ SPUTUM / LUNG

☐ ULTRASOUND   ☐ OTHER

INTERDISCIPLINARY ROUNDS

TODAY'S EXERCISES

☐ RANGE OF MOTION   ☐ SIT IN CHAIR

☐ REPOSITIONING   ☐ BICYCLE ·

☐ SIT AT BEDSIDE   ☐ WALKING

☐ STAND AT BEDSIDE   ☐ BEDREST

WHAT ARE THE MAJOR ISSUES / CONCERNS TODAY? IS THE PATIENT GETTING BETTER OR WORSE? WHAT ARE SHORT- & LONG-TERM GOALS?

....

....

....

TODAY YOU (PATIENT) FELT:

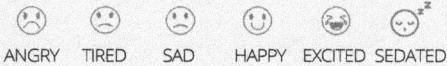

😠   😫   🙁   🙂   😆   😴
ANGRY   TIRED   SAD   HAPPY   EXCITED   SEDATED

BECAUSE: ☐ OTHER

1. ....

2. ....

3. ....

TODAY I (CAREGIVER) FELT:

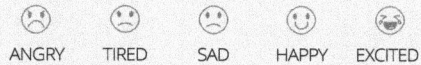

😠   😫   🙁   🙂   😆
ANGRY   TIRED   SAD   HAPPY   EXCITED

BECAUSE: ☐ OTHER

1. ....

2. ....

3. ....

WHAT HAPPENED TODAY?

PATIENT EVENTS | NEWS | MAJOR WORLD EVENTS | FAMILY EVENTS | VISITORS | ACTIVITIES | ICU ENVIRONMENT | SOUNDS | LIFE UPDATES | HOLIDAYS | RECOVERY MILESTONE

....

....

....

....

....

TODAY WE ARE GRATEFUL FOR...

1. ....

2. ....

3. ....

TODAY'S MESSAGE OF HOPE

....

....

....

....

QUOTE OF THE DAY

"For sleep, riches and health to be truly enjoyed, they must be interrupted." - Johann Paul Friedrich

TODAY'S ENTRY IS COMPLETED BY: ....

THERAPEUTIC
JOURNAL

TODAY'S DATE: ....

ROOM #: ....

ICU PHYSICIAN: ....

DAY NURSE: ....

NIGHT NURSE: ....

NUMBER OF IV PUMPS

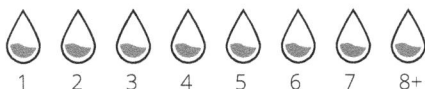

1   2   3   4   5   6   7   8+

IV LINES

☐ IV LINE   ☐ INTRAOSSEOUS

☐ CENTRAL LINE   ☐ PORT

☐ PICC LINE   ☐ OTHER

☐ DIALYSIS LINE

BREATHING SUPPORT

☐ INTUBATED   ☐ EXTUBATED

☐ VENTILATOR   ☐ HIGH FLOW

☐ TRACHEOSTOMY   ☐ NASAL PRONGS

☐ BIPAP / CPAP   ☐ ROOM AIR

☐ FACE MASK   ☐ OTHER

LEVEL OF CONSCIOUSNESS

☐ AWAKE   ☐ SEIZURE

☐ ALERT   ☐ AGITATED

☐ ORIENTED   ☐ HALLUCINATIONS

☐ PARALYTIC MEDICATION ☐ CONFUSED

☐ SEDATED   ☐ DELIRIOUS

☐ LETHARGIC   ☐ OTHER

NUTRITION

☐ NOTHING BY MOUTH   ☐ ICE CHIPS / CLEAR FLUIDS

☐ FEEDING TUBE   ☐ PUREED DIET

☐ FEEDS HELD   ☐ REGULAR

☐ TPN (IV)   ☐ OTHER

WOUNDS / INJURIES

....

....

DAILY PROGRESS AND GOALS

EACH DAY, THERE MAY BE ONE OR MORE GOALS OF CARE THAT THE TEAM IS HOPING THE PATIENT WILL ACHIEVE.

....

....

NOTES

....

....

....

TESTS PERFORMED TODAY

☐ X-RAY   ☐ BLOOD TESTS

☐ CT SCAN   ☐ BREATHING TRIAL

☐ MRI   ☐ SPUTUM / LUNG

☐ ULTRASOUND   ☐ OTHER

INTERDISCIPLINARY ROUNDS

TODAY'S EXERCISES

☐ RANGE OF MOTION   ☐ SIT IN CHAIR

☐ REPOSITIONING   ☐ BICYCLE

☐ SIT AT BEDSIDE   ☐ WALKING

☐ STAND AT BEDSIDE   ☐ BEDREST

WHAT ARE THE MAJOR ISSUES / CONCERNS TODAY? IS THE PATIENT GETTING BETTER OR WORSE? WHAT ARE SHORT- & LONG-TERM GOALS?

TODAY YOU (PATIENT) FELT:

ANGRY   TIRED   SAD   HAPPY   EXCITED   SEDATED

BECAUSE: ☐ OTHER

1.

2.

3.

TODAY I (CAREGIVER) FELT:

ANGRY   TIRED   SAD   HAPPY   EXCITED

BECAUSE: ☐ OTHER

1.

2.

3.

WHAT HAPPENED TODAY?

PATIENT EVENTS | NEWS | MAJOR WORLD EVENTS | FAMILY EVENTS | VISITORS | ACTIVITIES | ICU ENVIRONMENT | SOUNDS | LIFE UPDATES | HOLIDAYS | RECOVERY MILESTONE

TODAY WE ARE GRATEFUL FOR...

1.

2.

3.

TODAY'S MESSAGE OF HOPE

QUOTE OF THE DAY

"If you can't fly then run, if you can't run then walk, if you can't walk then crawl, but whatever you do you have to keep moving forward." - Martin Luther King Jr.

CARE TRANSITION TRACKER

S   M   T   W   T   F   S

JAN

FEB

MAR

APR

MAY

JUN

JUL

AUG

SEP

OCT

NOV

DEC

HOW TO USE THIS TRACKER

Patients are transferred frequently within hospitals and sometimes to other hospitals for specialized care or transitioning closer to home. Documenting this journey can be very helpful to piece together their experience. Record the date the patient was transferred and location(s) they were transferred to. You can include locations like ICU to the inpatient unit, to the operating room, for diagnostic imaging (MRI, CT), etc.

C A R E   T R A N S I T I O N   T R A C K E R

	S	M	T	W	T	F	S
JAN							
FEB							
MAR							
APR							
MAY							
JUN							
JUL							
AUG							
SEP							
OCT							
NOV							
DEC							

HOW TO USE THIS TRACKER

Patients are transferred frequently within hospitals and sometimes to other hospitals for specialized care or transitioning closer to home. Documenting this journey can be very helpful to piece together their experience. Record the date the patient was transferred and location(s) they were transferred to. You can include locations like ICU to the inpatient unit, to the operating room, for diagnostic imaging (MRI, CT), etc.

QUESTIONS
AND
PHYSICIAN
MEETINGS

THE **QUESTIONS** SECTION

An ICU experience naturally brings many questions for families. This section allows you to write your questions and take note of the answers you receive. It is highly encouraged to take notes as you may not realize how difficult it is to retain information while under immense stress. Documenting questions and answers here can also be helpful when the patient is ready to learn about their story.

DATE

DATE

QUESTIONS

DATE

DATE

DATE

QUESTIONS

DATE

DATE

DATE

QUESTIONS

DATE

DATE

DATE

QUESTIONS

DATE

DATE

DATE

QUESTIONS

DATE

DATE

DATE

PHYSICIAN **FAMILY** **CONFERENCE** MEETING NOTES

DATE

ATTENDEES: NEXT STEPS:

MEETING NOTES

PHYSICIAN **FAMILY** **CONFERENCE** MEETING NOTES

DATE

ATTENDEES:

NEXT STEPS:

MEETING NOTES

PHYSICIAN **FAMILY** **CONFERENCE** MEETING NOTES

DATE

ATTENDEES: NEXT STEPS:

MEETING NOTES

_____

_____

_____

_____

_____

_____

_____

_____

_____

_____

_____

_____

_____

PHYSICIAN **FAMILY** **CONFERENCE** MEETING NOTES

DATE

ATTENDEES:

NEXT STEPS:

MEETING NOTES

PHYSICIAN **FAMILY**
CONFERENCE MEETING NOTES

DATE

ATTENDEES: NEXT STEPS:

MEETING NOTES

....

....

....

....

....

....

....

....

....

....

....

....

....

....

....

....

PHYSICIAN **FAMILY** **CONFERENCE** MEETING NOTES

DATE

ATTENDEES:

NEXT STEPS:

MEETING NOTES

PHYSICIAN **FAMILY** **CONFERENCE** MEETING NOTES

DATE

ATTENDEES: NEXT STEPS:

MEETING NOTES

PHYSICIAN **FAMILY** **CONFERENCE** MEETING NOTES

DATE

ATTENDEES:

NEXT STEPS:

MEETING NOTES

PHYSICIAN **FAMILY**
CONFERENCE MEETING NOTES

DATE

ATTENDEES: NEXT STEPS:

MEETING NOTES

PHYSICIAN **FAMILY**
CONFERENCE MEETING NOTES

DATE

ATTENDEES:

NEXT STEPS:

MEETING NOTES

PHYSICIAN **FAMILY** **CONFERENCE** MEETING NOTES

DATE

ATTENDEES: NEXT STEPS:

MEETING NOTES

_____

_____

_____

_____

_____

_____

_____

_____

_____

_____

_____

_____

_____

_____

MESSAGES OF
LOVE
AND HOPE

MESSAGES FROM YOUR
FRIENDS AND FAMILY

MESSAGES FROM YOUR
FRIENDS AND FAMILY

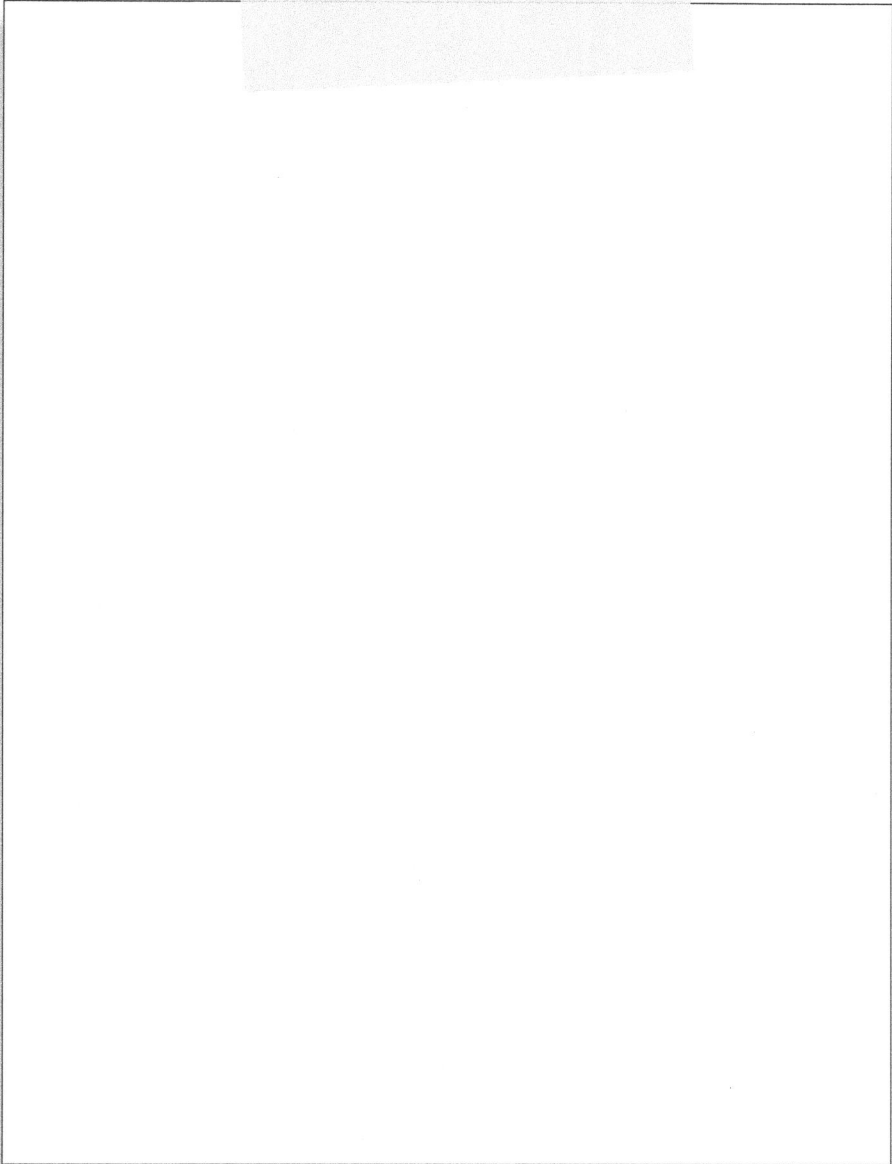

MESSAGES FROM YOUR
FRIENDS AND FAMILY

MESSAGES FROM YOUR
FRIENDS AND FAMILY

MESSAGES FROM YOUR
FRIENDS AND FAMILY

MESSAGES FROM YOUR
FRIENDS AND FAMILY

MESSAGES FROM YOUR
FRIENDS AND FAMILY

MESSAGES FROM YOUR
HEALTH CARE TEAM

MESSAGES FROM YOUR
HEALTH CARE TEAM

MESSAGES FROM YOUR
HEALTH CARE TEAM

MESSAGES FROM YOUR
HEALTH CARE TEAM

MESSAGES FROM YOUR
HEALTH CARE TEAM

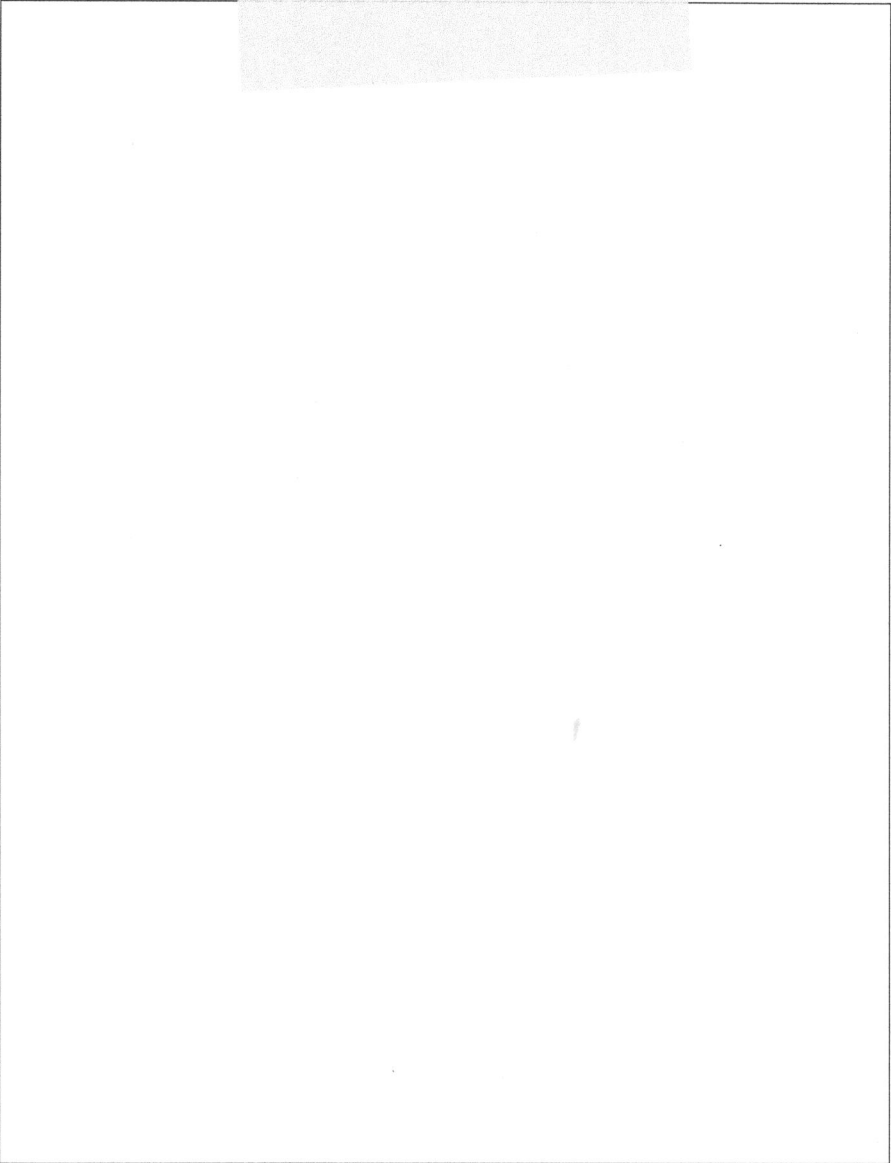

MESSAGES FROM YOUR
HEALTH CARE TEAM

PHOTOS

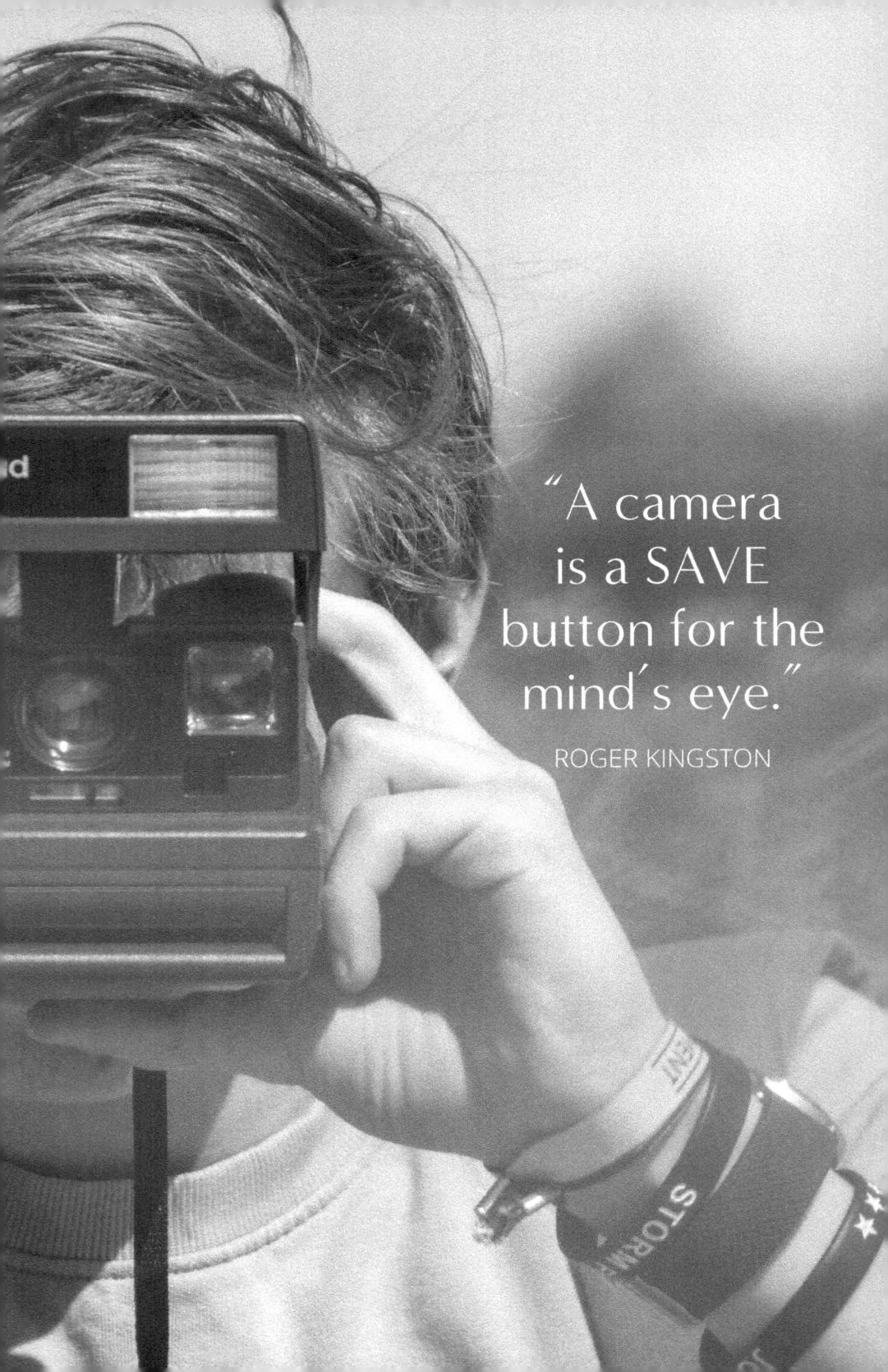

"A camera
is a SAVE
button for the
mind's eye."

ROGER KINGSTON

RECOVERY **MILESTONE** TRACKER

Going through a serious illness has many ups and downs. It's always easier for people to remember the bad days. This page is a reminder to celebrate the wins as patients get better!

DATE

.... FIRST TIME AWAKE

.... OXYGEN LOWERED

.... BREATHING TUBE OUT

.... FIRST ICE CHIPS

.... FIRST SIP OF WATER

.... FIRST TIME SITTING UP

.... FIRST TIME STANDING

.... FIRST STEPS

.... FIRST HUGS FROM FAMILY

.... FIRST REUNION

.... TRANSFER OUT OF ICU

.... DISCHARGE DAY

Adhere polaroids here
5.4 cm x 8.6 cm

Adhere polaroids here
5.4 cm x 8.6 cm

Adhere polaroids here
5.4 cm x 8.6 cm

Adhere polaroids here
5.4 cm x 8.6 cm

Adhere polaroids here
5.4 cm x 8.6 cm

Adhere polaroids here
5.4 cm x 8.6 cm

Adhere polaroids here
5.4 cm x 8.6 cm

Adhere polaroids here
5.4 cm x 8.6 cm

Adhere polaroids here
5.4 cm x 8.6 cm

Adhere polaroids here
5.4 cm x 8.6 cm

Adhere polaroids here
5.4 cm x 8.6 cm

Adhere polaroids here
5.4 cm x 8.6 cm

Adhere polaroids here
5.4 cm x 8.6 cm

Adhere polaroids here
5.4 cm x 8.6 cm

Adhere polaroids here
5.4 cm x 8.6 cm

Adhere polaroids here
5.4 cm x 8.6 cm

POWER OF ATTORNEY & DECISION-MAKER RESOURCES

CONTACT LIST

- NAME
- PHONE
- EMAIL
- WEBSITE
- ADDRESS
- NOTES

- NAME
- PHONE
- EMAIL
- WEBSITE
- ADDRESS
- NOTES

- NAME
- PHONE
- EMAIL
- WEBSITE
- ADDRESS
- NOTES

- NAME
- PHONE
- EMAIL
- WEBSITE
- ADDRESS
- NOTES

- NAME
- PHONE
- EMAIL
- WEBSITE
- ADDRESS
- NOTES

- NAME
- PHONE
- EMAIL
- WEBSITE
- ADDRESS
- NOTES

- NAME
- PHONE
- EMAIL
- WEBSITE
- ADDRESS
- NOTES

- NAME
- PHONE
- EMAIL
- WEBSITE
- ADDRESS
- NOTES

- NAME
- PHONE
- EMAIL
- WEBSITE
- ADDRESS
- NOTES

- NAME
- PHONE
- EMAIL
- WEBSITE
- ADDRESS
- NOTES

CONTACT LIST

👤 NAME	👤 NAME
📞 PHONE	📞 PHONE
✉ EMAIL	✉ EMAIL
🌐 WEBSITE	🌐 WEBSITE
📍 ADDRESS	📍 ADDRESS
📋 NOTES	📋 NOTES
👤 NAME	👤 NAME
📞 PHONE	📞 PHONE
✉ EMAIL	✉ EMAIL
🌐 WEBSITE	🌐 WEBSITE
📍 ADDRESS	📍 ADDRESS
📋 NOTES	📋 NOTES
👤 NAME	👤 NAME
📞 PHONE	📞 PHONE
✉ EMAIL	✉ EMAIL
🌐 WEBSITE	🌐 WEBSITE
📍 ADDRESS	📍 ADDRESS
📋 NOTES	📋 NOTES
👤 NAME	👤 NAME
📞 PHONE	📞 PHONE
✉ EMAIL	✉ EMAIL
🌐 WEBSITE	🌐 WEBSITE
📍 ADDRESS	📍 ADDRESS
📋 NOTES	📋 NOTES
👤 NAME	👤 NAME
📞 PHONE	📞 PHONE
✉ EMAIL	✉ EMAIL
🌐 WEBSITE	🌐 WEBSITE
📍 ADDRESS	📍 ADDRESS
📋 NOTES	📋 NOTES

CONTACT LIST

- NAME
- PHONE
- EMAIL
- WEBSITE
- ADDRESS
- NOTES

- NAME
- PHONE
- EMAIL
- WEBSITE
- ADDRESS
- NOTES

- NAME
- PHONE
- EMAIL
- WEBSITE
- ADDRESS
- NOTES

- NAME
- PHONE
- EMAIL
- WEBSITE
- ADDRESS
- NOTES

- NAME
- PHONE
- EMAIL
- WEBSITE
- ADDRESS
- NOTES

- NAME
- PHONE
- EMAIL
- WEBSITE
- ADDRESS
- NOTES

- NAME
- PHONE
- EMAIL
- WEBSITE
- ADDRESS
- NOTES

- NAME
- PHONE
- EMAIL
- WEBSITE
- ADDRESS
- NOTES

- NAME
- PHONE
- EMAIL
- WEBSITE
- ADDRESS
- NOTES

- NAME
- PHONE
- EMAIL
- WEBSITE
- ADDRESS
- NOTES

THE **HOSPITAL** CHECKLIST

BRING TO THE HOSPITAL

- [ ] Health card (check expiry date)
- [ ] Advance care plan / directives
- [ ] Hearing aids (and batteries)
- [ ] Eyeglasses
- [ ] Dentures
- [ ] Toiletries
- [ ] Pictures and cards
- [ ] Notebook
- [ ] Important contacts list
- [ ] Personal CPAP machine

- [ ] Health insurance documents
- [ ] Electric shaver
- [ ] Footwear with grip
- [ ] Phone charger
- [ ] Most recent list of prescriptions
- [ ] Patient name labels
- [ ] Power of Attorney documents
- [ ] Immunization records
- [ ] Entertainment (e.g., books, magazine, device)
- [ ]

LEAVE AT HOME

- [ ] Flowers
- [ ] Personal linens
- [ ] Valuables (e.g. wedding bands)
- [ ] Wallet

- [ ] Young children under 3
- [ ] Large bulky items
- [ ] Will * Ensure it can be located by the patient's executor
- [ ]

INPATIENT UNIT (OR EXTUBATED IN ICU)

- [ ] Robe
- [ ] Slippers / shoes with grip
- [ ] Accessibility aids
- [ ] Mobility aids

- [ ] Phone charger
- [ ]
- [ ]
- [ ]

- [ ] Due to high risk of loss and theft in hospitals, leave these items home if the patient is sedated / unconscious. Bring in when the patient begins to wake up or when the care team asks for them.

IMPORTANT INFORMATION
FOR POA
BANKING AND BILLING INFORMATION

Use this sheet to identify if there are any outstanding debts or required payments to look after while the patient is critically ill.

BANKING INSTITUTION _____

_____

CREDIT CARD 1 _____

CREDIT CARD 2 _____

CREDIT CARD 3 _____

CREDIT CARD 4 _____

LOAN 1 _____

LOAN 2 _____

MORTGAGE DUE _____

RENT DUE _____

DOES THE PATIENT OWE CHILD OR
SPOUSAL SUPPORT PAYMENTS?   YES   NO   UNSURE

LINE OF CREDIT _____

AUTO PAYMENT _____

STUDENT LOAN _____

BUSINESS LOAN _____

LEASED ASSETS _____

ACCRUED EXPENSES _____

OTHER DEBTS? _____

IMPORTANT INFORMATION
FOR POA
BANKING AND BILLING INFORMATION

Use this sheet to identify if there are any outstanding debts or required payments to look after while the patient is critically ill.

TELEPHONE ....

....

CELLPHONE ....

UTILITIES ....

TELEVISION ....

INTERNET ....

LIFE INSURANCE ....

HEALTH INSURANCE ....

HOME INSURANCE ....

....

LINE OF CREDIT ....

LINE OF CREDIT ....

LINE OF CREDIT ....

AUTO PAYMENT ....

STUDENT LOAN ....

BUSINESS LOAN ....

LEASED ASSETS ....

....

PROPERTY TAXES ....

IMPORTANT INFORMATION
FOR POA
BANKING AND BILLING INFORMATION

Use this sheet to identify if there are any outstanding debts or required payments to look after while the patient is critically ill.

Does the patient have the following documents?	Will - Public / Private Trust	POA - Personal Care POA - Property	Advance care plan Advance directives
ESTATE LAWYER			
BUSINESS LAWYER			
BOOKKEEPER			
ACCOUNTANT			
FAMILY DOCTOR			
INSURANCE REP			
FINANCIAL ADVISOR			
EMPLOYER			
MORTGAGE DUE			

SERVICES TO CONSIDER PAUSING DURING CRITICAL ILLNESS

MORTGAGE DUE	CELLULAR SERVICE	MEAL DELIVERY SERVICES
MAGAZINES	UPCOMING TRAVEL	TECH SUBSCRIPTIONS
NEWSPAPERS	SOFTWARE SUBSCRIPTIONS	GROOMING SUBSCRIPTIONS
GYM MEMBERSHIPS	MEMBERSHIPS (e.g., CLUBS, MUSEUMS)	STREAMING SERVICE (TV / MUSIC)

SERVICES REQUIRING ACTION DURING CRITICAL ILLNESS

PROFESSIONAL LICENSE RENEWALS	UTILITY BILLS
PATIENT'S HEALTH CARD EXPIRATION	DAYCARE / CHILDCARE
MORTGAGE PAYMENTS	PHONE
CREDIT CARD MINIMUM PAYMENTS	LOAN PAYMENTS
TAX PAYMENTS	PET CARE / GROOMING

INSURANCE POLICIES: AUTO | HOME | COTTAGE | BUSINESS | ILLNESS | LIFE

PASSWORD MANAGER

FOR THE POWER OF ATTORNEY FOR PERSONAL CARE AND / OR PROPERTY

WEBSITE
USERNAME
PASSWORD
NOTES

WEBSITE
USERNAME
PASSWORD
NOTES

WEBSITE
USERNAME
PASSWORD
NOTES

WEBSITE
USERNAME
PASSWORD
NOTES

WEBSITE
USERNAME
PASSWORD
NOTES

WEBSITE
USERNAME
PASSWORD
NOTES

WEBSITE
USERNAME
PASSWORD
NOTES

WEBSITE
USERNAME
PASSWORD
NOTES

WEBSITE
USERNAME
PASSWORD
NOTES

WEBSITE
USERNAME
PASSWORD
NOTES

WEBSITE
USERNAME
PASSWORD
NOTES

WEBSITE
USERNAME
PASSWORD
NOTES

WEBSITE
USERNAME
PASSWORD
NOTES

WEBSITE
USERNAME
PASSWORD
NOTES

IMPORTANT INFORMATION
FOR POA

SMALL BUSINESS DETAILS

Is the patient a small business owner?

YES   **NO**

If **yes**, here are few helpful questions to guide management of the business while the patient is unwell.

How critical is the founder's role in the day-to-day operations?

Are there any Standard Operating Procedures, Training Manuals or key personnel that can be relied on?

Are there any legal or contractual obligations or liabilities that require immediate action?

Is there a business partner or key personnel for key decision-making and leadership?

Who has access to and control over the business' financial accounts?

Are there employees that need to be paid? Who looks after this?

Is there a business legacy plan in place outlining steps in emergencies?

Is there illness insurance or savings to support loss of income?

Does messaging need to be sent to employees, clients or business partners regarding the state of health of the founder? Is this in alignment with the business strategy and brand? Could this hurt the business?

Consider privacy protection in the message strategy.

IMPORTANT INFORMATION
FOR POA
SMALL BUSINESS DETAILS

This section is designed to help family members gather information to operationalize a business in the absence of a business plan, Standard Operating Procedure or Legacy Plan.

BUSINESS NAME ....

CO-FOUNDER NAME ....

CO-FOUNDER CONTACT ....

BOOKKEEPER ....

ACCOUNTANT ....

BUSINESS # ....

CRA ACCOUNT INFO ....

BUSINESS YEAR-END ....

LEGAL STRUCTURE   Sole proprietorship   Partnership
                      LLC   Corporation

RENT / LOANS DUE ....

TAX INSTALLMENTS DUE ....

PASSWORD MANAGER ....

BUSINESS OPERATIONS PLATFORMS / TECH STACK

AIRBNB	HI5	PINTEREST	TIKTOK
BEHANCE	KUAISHOU	QQ	TUMBLR
CLIENT RELATION MANAGER	LINE	QUORA	TWITCH
	LINKEDIN	REDDIT	TWITTER | X
DISCORD	MASTODON	RENREN	VERO
DOUBAN	MEWE	SIGNAL	VIMEO
DRIBBBLE	MEDIUM	SINA WEIBO	VINE
DUBSADO	MEETUP	SHOPIFY	VRBO
ELLO	MIX	SLACK	WECHAT
ETSY	MYSPACE	SNAPCHAT	WHATSAPP
FACEBOOK	NEXTDOOR	STUMBLE UPON	YAHOO GROUPS
FIVERR	ORKUT	SWARM	YELP
FLICKR	PATH	THREADS	YOUTUBE
FOURSQUARE	PEACH	THRIVECART	OTHER
GOOGLE+	PERISCOPE	INSTAGRAM	

BUSINESS EMAIL

GMAIL
HUSHMAIL
OUTLOOK
YAHOO MAIL
APPLE MAIL
AOL MAIL
OTHER

BOOKKEEPING

QUICKBOOKS
WAVE
ZERO
OTHER

THINGS TO DO AFTER YOU
LEAVE THE HOSPITAL

☐ If you're able, **come back to visit** the ICU. Staff love to see how well their patients are doing. If it's too hard to come in (emotionally or physically), send a letter, a card or video message.

☐ Critical illness is very hard on the body and the patient will feel very weak due to muscle loss. **Physical therapy and rehabilitation programs** are essential for long-term recovery.

☐ Surviving a critical illness is an incredible gift but often leaves behind psychological trauma. **Counseling for post-traumatic stress injury** (PTSI) and post-intensive care syndrome (PICS) is highly encouraged for both patients and loved ones to help process their experiences. See if your hospital has an ICU follow-up clinic.

☐ **Healing takes time** and is a long-term process. Be patient and accepting of the range of emotions you and your family might experience. Seek professional help with navigating these emotions.

☐ **Lean on family and friends** for support during your / your loved one's recovery.

☐ Prepare your power of attorney or decision-makers for future health directives with **advance care planning.**

☐ **Get your legal affairs and estate in order.**

☐ If you had a good experience, **let the clinical manager know.** Health care providers pour their blood, sweat and tears into their patients. Acknowledgment for their hard work boosts morale on nursing teams and is one of the best gifts a nurse can get. And it's FREE!

GRIEF, LOSS
AND END-OF-LIFE
RESOURCES

UNDERSTANDING
GRIEF & LOSS

WHAT IS GRIEF?

Grief is a very complicated feeling and presents itself in different ways. People think grief only comes when someone has died. Grief can begin at any stage of illness and recovery. It can also occur if the patient is not in serious danger but has been diagnosed with a serious illness with a poor outcome (e.g., Stage 4 cancer). Grief is the emotional feelings that accompany loss (Oates & Maani-Fogelman, 2022).

WHAT DOES GRIEF LOOK LIKE IN ICU?

Grief can express itself in different ways when a loved one is critically ill. It may present as:

- Infighting between families leading to relationship breakdown and added stress
- Denial or non-acceptance of a particular prognosis or diagnosis
- Conflict with the care team
- Feeling distrust with the care team (often resolved by more communication)
- Anger is often the first emotion that presents with grief
- Avoidance—family avoiding coming in to visit with their loved one
- A sense of cognitive overload or brain fog
- Having trouble processing information
- Physical symptoms: feeling anxious, hungry / not hungry, insomnia, headaches, fatigue
- Blame
- Feeling helpless
- Irritability
- Difficulty concentrating
- Difficulty sleeping
- These are some examples—there are many other unique presentations

STAGES OF **GRIEF**

A NOTE ABOUT GRIEF AND LOSS

The following descriptions of grief and loss were perfectly described by Oates, J. & Maani-Fogelman, P.A. (2022). *Nursing grief and loss*. StatPearls Publishing. All credit goes to these authors for their excellent explanations. To learn more, please reference the full text of their paper.

While these stages are presented in a sequential order, it is important to know many people experience grief in a unique sequence, which may be out of order of what is described below. Individuals may also enter two stages at the same time.

Grief is a very unique experience and different for every person and family. Please lean on your care team for support.

If you wish to learn more about grief, use this QR code to access MyGrief. ca. This website offers modules to help you understand your own grief and learn about the grieving process.

There are 28 modules that speak to numerous topics including:

- Anticipatory grief
- Self-care
- Loss of a spouse
- Loss of a parent
- Loss of a child
- Pregnancy loss
- Loss of a sibling
- Loss of a grandparent
- Loss of a friend or co-worker
- Illness progression
- MAiD
- 2SLGBTQ+

Reference: Oates, J. & Maani-Fogelman, P.A. (2022). *Nursing grief and loss*. StatPearls Publishing.

STAGES OF **GRIEF**

SHOCK

When a person or family learns about a serious illness, approaching end of life or death for the first time, they may enter a state of shock. This can present as appearing numb, not able to process the information provided and potentially asking the same question(s) repeatedly. Oates and Maani-Fogelman (2022) state entering shock may be a protective mechanism that prevents the person from immediate emotional overwhelm.

ANGER

The stage of denial may bring on many emotions, including feeling like their new world has no meaning as a result of the loss of a loved one. Their life may feel very overwhelming. They may struggle to make sense of their new life. The feeling of numbness may continue as a protective mechanism. While the stage of denial was once limited to denying the loss took place, the definition includes the person may deny their own experience of their feelings (Oates & Maani-Fogelman, 2022). As an individual is able to accept that this loss is their reality, they will be able to move into the healing process and denial will begin to diminish (Oates & Maani-Fogelman, 2022).

DENIAL

Anger is a very common experience in the intensive care unit, where many families express frustration or anger about their loved one's illness experience. Oates and Maani-Fogelman (2022) say feeling and addressing anger is part of the healing and grieving process. They also encourage health care providers to recognize this as a demonstration of grief and pain and to not take outbursts and attacks personally (Oates & Maani-Fogelman, 2022).

Reference: Oates, J. & Maani-Fogelman, P.A. (2022). *Nursing grief and loss*. StatPearls Publishing.

STAGES OF **GRIEF**

BARGAINING

Oates and Maani-Fogelman (2022) explain bargaining may come in the form of "what if" statements.
- What if we found the cancer sooner?
- What if this accident never happened?

This questioning is common in grief and suggests the person wants life to return to how it was (Oates & Maani-Fogelman, 2022). Guilt often accompanies bargaining (Oates & Maani-Fogelman, 2022) where the person wishes they could have done something to change the outcome.

DEPRESSION

Depression in the context of a significant negative life event is not the same as depression as a mental illness. In this stage, depression is "an appropriate response to a significant loss" (Oates & Maani-Fogelman, 2022). It may take time for the person to realize the loss is permanent, and once this is realized, symptoms of depression may set in. Symptoms may include not engaging with friends, changes in activities that make the person happy or intense sadness (Oates & Maani-Fogelman, 2022). While many people choose to navigate their feelings privately, it is always encouraged to seek the help of grief counselors and professionals. This recommendation is even stronger when the loss is unexpected (like that of a loved one in intensive care).

Self-care and listening to what the body is saying is very important during this time. If you or someone you know is feeling depressed, this is the body saying it needs "deep rest." Try to take the time needed to sleep, eat, take time off work, arrange support for child care, eat take-out or other premade meals to lighten the load and make room for healing.

Remember: Depressed = "Deep rest"

Reference: Oates, J. & Maani-Fogelman, P.A. (2022). *Nursing grief and loss*. StatPearls Publishing.

STAGES OF **GRIEF**

TESTING

As people learn to navigate their new life following loss, they may change careers or try new things that feel right in that new phase of life. It is a phase of exploration as they try and make sense of their new world (Oates & Maani-Fogelman, 2022).

ACCEPTANCE

The stage of acceptance allows for the individual to accept the reality for what it is, and realizing it is permanant (Oates & Maani-Fogelman, 2022). There may be some days that are emotionally challenging but the individual will return to navigating life (Oates & Maani-Fogelman, 2022). Radical acceptance is a form of behavioral therapy that helps people accept the challenges of life that may be of interest as one moves through their grief healing.

DEFINING LOSS

For many, loss represents someone who has died. The feelings of grief and loss can also be felt when death has not occurred.

Loss can also refer to:

- The loss of a physical ability (e.g., losing one's ability to see or walk)
- The loss of one's sense of health (e.g., diagnosed with a serious heart condition)
- Missing the anticipated birth of a baby
- Loss of control or feelings of helplessness when a loved one is in ICU
- Loss of support from a partner (e.g., parent of young children feeling overwhelmed by moving into the default parent role)

Reference: Oates, J. & Maani-Fogelman, P.A. (2022). *Nursing grief and loss*. StatPearls Publishing.

WHAT TO DO WHEN
YOUR LOVED ONE **MIGHT DIE**

If you are reading this section, firstly please accept our most sincere condolences. Losing a loved one (un)expectedly is tragic and painful. This is an experience you will always remember and finding ways to honor your loved one may help to ease these memories following the experience.

Notify close friends and family.

Facilitate plans to spend time with your loved one (e.g., notify your work; make child care arrangements).

Social work can provide a letter for work or travel as needed.

Create a peaceful environment in the hospital room.
- Fill the room with music.
- Print out photos.
- Bring a blanket from home.

You may wish to provide personal care like brushing their hair or painting their nails.

Start thinking about what arrangements you might need to take following your loved one's death (e.g., funeral, cremation). This may be a good discussion to have among family.

Ask the health care team to notify spiritual care to provide prayers, blessings or emotional and spiritual support.

Understand all the ways the ICU team will ensure your loved one will be kept comfortable during the end-of-life process.

Have an open discussion about what the dying process might look like.

WHAT TO DO WHEN
YOUR LOVED ONE **MIGHT DIE**

If children are involved, have early discussions about the illness, providing age appropriate explanations of the state of their loved one's illness and the reality that they might die.

This resource (scan QR code) helps to educate and help start discussions around death and dying with children.

Notify the executor named in your loved one's will and ensure they can locate the original will.

Allow yourself to grieve and feel all your feelings. Self-care is very important during this time.

Review life insurance documents.

Attempt to determine the patient's wishes for organ donation. You may initiate this conversation with the care team.

WHAT TO DO WHEN
YOUR LOVED ONE **HAS DIED**

If you are reading this section, firstly please accept our most sincere condolences.
Losing a loved one (un)expectedly is tragic and painful.

Spend as much time with your loved one in ICU after they have passed as you need.

Notify close friends and family.

Consider what arrangements you might like to make for your loved one's remains:
Funeral home
Direct cremation
Full body donation to science

Look after care of dependents (e.g., children), pets and the well-being of grieving family members.

Ensure the patient's personal property (e.g., home) is being monitored, maintained and taken care of.

Take time to grieve before initiating the funeral arrangement process.

Consider grief support services in the form of 1:1 counseling or support groups to help process your loss.

WHAT TO DO WHEN YOUR LOVED ONE **HAS DIED**

Contact a spiritual leader in the community who you may want to be part of arrangements.

Continue talking about your loved one and the memories you hold.

Take home any valuables and belongings (e.g., identification, jewelry, electronics, photos, clothing, personal items). If they were admitted from an inpatient area, be sure to check that area for belongings as well.

Obtain a letter confirming death from the funeral home to begin managing affairs without the formal death certificate.

Notify the executor named in your loved one's will that they have passed so the executor may initiate estate proceedings.

Here is a link to obtain a death certificate in the province of Ontario. Remember to order many copies as there will be several requests for them.

WHAT TO DO WHEN YOUR LOVED ONE **HAS DIED**

These are a few links to assist families in Ontario specifically to help them get started with settling their deceased loved one's affairs. You can find similar resources for your province or state online.

Use this QR code resource from the **Province of Ontario** to learn how to apply for probate of an estate.

Use this QR code resource from the **Province of Ontario** to help with your next steps on what to do when someone dies.

Use this QR code resource from the **Government of Canada** to help with your next steps on how to notify the federal government of a death.

FOR THOSE USING THIS JOURNAL OUTSIDE OF CANADA:

Your ICU care team may have a social worker or other clinical leader who might help you find similar resources and direction in your country.

ORDERING **A DEATH CERTIFICATE** IN CANADA

Hospitals do not provide the death certificate. A death certificate must be obtained from the Ministry of Health though the province. Use the following QR codes to quickly access provincial and territorial resources for obtaining a death certificate.

ALBERTA

BRITISH COLUMBIA

MANITOBA

NEW BRUNSWICK

NEWFOUNDLAND & LABRADOR

NORTHWEST TERRITORIES

NOVA SCOTIA

NUNAVUT

PRINCE EDWARD ISLAND

QUEBEC

SASKATCHEWAN

YUKON

NOTE: These QR codes were verified as functional at the time of their creation. However, their functionality may no longer be guaranteed.

Transitioning from the hospital back home
is a big step. This leaves families and patients
feeling very vulnerable and uncertain.

ACE Planning Company exists
to provide support and peace of mind
during this challenging transition.

| EDUCATION | PLANNING | SYSTEM NAVIGATION | SUPPORT |

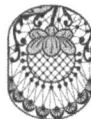

ADVANCE CARE &
EMERGENCY PLANNING COMPANY

PLAN FOR THE (UN)EXPECTED

LET'S CONNECT

(365) 228-7167

carly@aceplannningco.com

www.aceplanningco.com

CONTRIBUTING SUBJECT MATTER **EXPERTS**

ACE Planning Company would like to acknowledge the experts who took time to review this guide and provide feedback. If you need assistance navigating your loved one's care or personal experience, please reach out to these professionals.

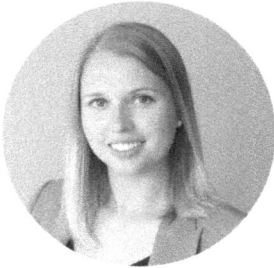

Anouck van Balen Walter, LLP

Estate planning, dispute resolution
and notary services
vBW Law
anouck@vbwlaw.ca

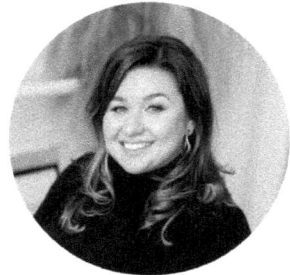

Elena Favaro Viana, LLP

Lawyer for Entrepreneurs and Small
Businesses
EFV Legal
hello@elenafavaroviana.com

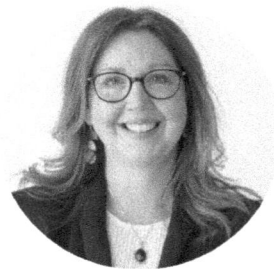

Stephanie Rackus

Psychotherapist (Qualifying)
and ICU Registered Nurse
Connect with Stephanie
stephanie.rackus.ocp@gmail.com

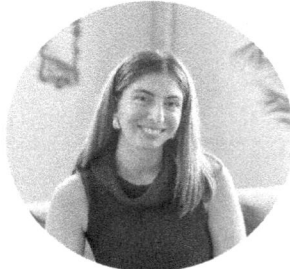

Ivana Di Cosola

Registered Social Worker
and Psychotherapist
Innerbloom Therapy
info@innerbloomtherapy.ca

Are you interested in implementing ICU journals in your ICU?

INCOME STREAM FOR YOUR UNIT: Selling these journals to families could be a great way for nursing unit councils or teams to earn extra income.

We can help with:

- Wholesale / bulk purchase pricing
- Community journal bundle sponsorship programs
- Staff onboarding support—on-site (GTA) or virtual education
- Learning videos for staff
- Email support for families
- Organizational templates including:
  - Email to onboard families to using the ICU journal
  - Organizational policy templates that can be customized for your institution
- Would you like other learning materials? Let's see what we can do for you.

OR would you like these available in your hospital gift shop for patients and families to purchase?

Let's connect!
hello@aceplanningco.com

TO-DO LIST

- [ ] ....
- [ ] ....
- [ ] ....
- [ ] ....
- [ ] ....
- [ ] ....
- [ ] ....
- [ ] ....
- [ ] ....
- [ ] ....
- [ ] ....
- [ ] ....
- [ ] ....
- [ ] ....
- [ ] ....
- [ ] ....
- [ ] ....
- [ ] ....

TO-DO LIST

- [ ] ....
- [ ] ....
- [ ] ....
- [ ] ....
- [ ] ....
- [ ] ....
- [ ] ....
- [ ] ....
- [ ] ....
- [ ] ....
- [ ] ....
- [ ] ....
- [ ] ....
- [ ] ....
- [ ] ....
- [ ] ....
- [ ] ....
- [ ] ....

NOTES

NOTES

NOTES

NOTES

NOTES

SOCIAL MEDIA

Follow along with ACE Planning Company

FACEBOOK | INSTAGRAM | TIK TOK | YOUTUBE | THREADS | X / TWITTER | LINKEDIN

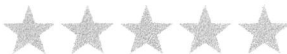

ACE Planning Company

@aceplanningco

@aceplanningco

@aceplanningco

@aceplanningco

@aceplanningco

Carly Hickey

RELATABLE CONTENT

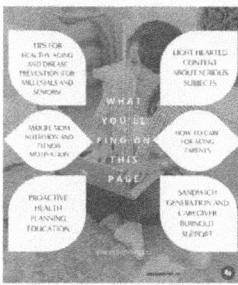

aceplanningco

Carly RN (NP student) | Proactive Healthcare Planner

361 Posts   1,395 Followers   1,098 Following

104

Show all comments (17)

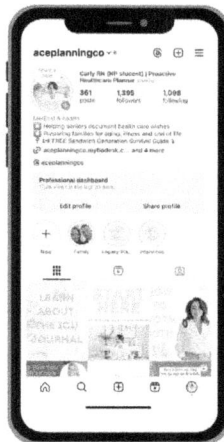

EDUCATIONAL CONTENT

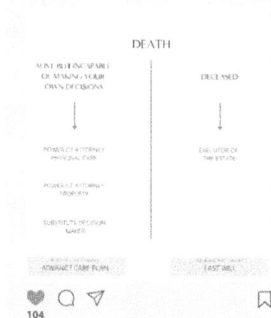

DEATH

104

Show all comments (17)

carly@aceplanningco.com | www.aceplanningco.com | (365) 228-7167

PLEASE
REVIEW US ON

Google

★★★★★

ACE Planning Company

SCAN HERE

WE WANT TO HEAR
FROM YOU!

REVIEWS GO A LONG WAY TO SUPPORT
BUSINESSES. PLEASE TAKE A MINUTE TO
REVIEW US ON

Google

fEMPOWER
PUBLICATIONS

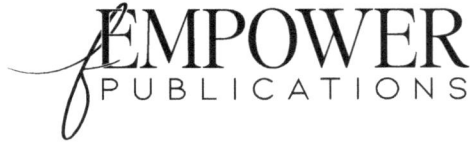

At fEMPOWER Publications,
we don't just publish books—we amplify movements.

We support thought leaders, visionary storytellers, and creative entrepreneurs
in transforming their ideas into powerful nonfiction books, journals, workbooks,
affirmation decks, and personal growth tools that leave lasting impact.

Our mission is to help our authors protect their soul's work, expand HER platform
beyond the page, and turn HER message into a timeless legacy.

www.fempower.pub | @fempower.pub ⬚

www.ingramcontent.com/pod-product-compliance
Lightning Source LLC
Chambersburg PA
CBHW040923210326
41597CB00030B/5156